THE ULTIMATE GUIDE TO INTERMITTENT FASTING FOR WOMEN OVER 50

TRANSFORM YOUR HEALTH: LOSE WEIGHT, DELAY AGING, INCREASE ENERGY, IMPROVE HEALTH, AND ENJOY LIFE

KEVIN STERLING

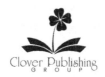

Clover Publishing
G R O U P

TABLE OF CONTENTS

INTRODUCTION

 Aging is not an option, not for anyone. It is how gracefully we handle the process and how lucky we are, as the process handles us. –

— CINDY MCDONALD

A long life should be one to celebrate. With a long life comes age, a nonnegotiable and inevitable aspect of who we are. It's something that signifies decades of joy, achievement, and growth, showing that we have so much to be proud of and thankful for. But unfortunately, many individuals, and women especially, miss out on the opportunity to truly relish in the wonders of living a long life. Many people believe that with age comes less beauty, less vitality, and less strength—a bias that can prove challenging for any woman who is trying to embrace age with grace.

And to an extent, the challenges that come with age are more than understandable. As an aging woman, you might be torn—you're worrying about whether people still care about or remember you as you approach this stage in your life. What's more is that your body is changing in dynamic ways as well, with menopause bringing about countless symptoms that put a damper on your day. Beyond that, you're probably frightened when thinking about your health—how is your health going to stand up to age? And that's not even to mention weight management.

Whatever you're struggling with as you age and change, it's valid and nothing to be ashamed of. Millions of women world-wide feel just like you do, meaning that you're far from alone in this battle. The way we perceive age has been shaped by societal norms and beauty standards, which means that the unrealistic expectations of beauty and age pushed upon you—and every woman—can make it all but impossible to love yourself with age. The fact of the matter is that these struggles aren't your fault!

Amidst all of this, I have some good news for you: You don't have to deal with these struggles alone or in confusion. There is one solution that can lessen the blow of every single one of the problems you're experiencing from age and social pressures: intermittent fasting. And lucky for you, this book contains every single secret to successful intermittent fasting for women over the age of 50. Intermittent fasting isn't a magical solution to aging, but it can certainly work some magic when it comes to alleviating menopausal symptoms, aiding in weight management, and so much more.

To make things even better, understanding intermittent fasting has never been easier! Within this book, you will unveil a one-of-a-kind, F.A.S.T. framework, serving as a comprehensive guide to helping you navigate intermittent fasting with ease and success:

- **Foundations of intermittent fasting:** The foundations of intermittent fasting, including what it is, how it works, and other basic facets of the concept that will drive you to success.
- **Aging and nutrition:** Unparalleled strategies for adopting the general principles of intermittent fasting, all specific to your unique stage of life.
- **Strategic planning and integration:** The keys to planning your fasting strategy, managing weight, and incorporating exercise—all based on your unique intermittent fasting plan.
- **Total wellness:** An expansion of intermittent fasting to include mental well-being strategies, long-term lifestyle changes, and holistic wellness.

Rest assured, it is never too late to take control of your health and start embracing a healthier lifestyle. In fact, the changes that you make from today forward can overshadow any health mistakes of the past—within reason—to help you live out the rest of your life with proactive strategies and success.

Imagine it: You wake up and feel better than ever. Full of energy, you're ready to start your day. You're confident and assured, feeling like yourself within your body. In fact, you know that there is nothing to be ashamed of! You can success-fully manage your weight, menopause symptoms, and other aspects of your health, and you know now that aging is a gift—not a curse. What could be more perfect than living the rest of life with this mindset?

If that's not enough to convince you, allow me to tell you a bit about myself. My name is Kevin Sterling. And while I could never connect to the experiences of being a woman over 50, I have certainly had my fair share of health struggles. I adore cooking. It's one of my favorite things to do, but it also contributed to my biggest nightmare. I've always loved exploring how food shapes others, but one day, it shaped me for the worst—I was diagnosed with prediabetes.

Prediabetes is no joke, and it runs in my family as well. It was on that day that I decided to make a change in how I interacted with food, my beloved hobby. I dived deep into the world of health and nutrition and found intermittent fasting. It is because of my experiences, my years of research (including research on how intermittent fasting impacts women), and my personal successes that this book is being brought to you today. I know first-hand just how valuable intermittent fasting can be!

My story isn't just about food; it's about empowerment, resilience, and the joy of positive change. Through this book, I hope to inspire you to venture toward happiness while consid-ering both food and age to be friends—not the enemy.

With that being said, you don't have to live in fear of aging. It is *never* too late to start taking care of yourself and transforming your health. If you commit to it right here and right now, you won't regret it. It's time to turn the page to a new chapter in your life, using your upcoming discoveries to understand how intermittent fasting can transform your health and perspective on aging, leading you to a happier and healthier life.

PART I

FOUNDATIONS OF INTERMITTENT FASTING

1

THE IF PRIMER—EMBRACING THE BASICS OF INTERMITTENT FASTING

Fasting is the single greatest natural healing therapy. It is nature's ancient, universal "remedy" for many problems.

— ELSON HAAS, M.D.

Before you can dig into a journey, it's important to understand the journey itself. In other words, in order for your intermittent fasting journey to be a success, it's important to understand what fasting is, why intermittent fasting works, and more, laying a solid foundation for your adventure with intermittent fasting. And that's just what this chapter helps you accomplish. By the end of this chapter, you'll have a firm understanding of intermittent fasting as the foundation for your experience. Let's dive in!

THE SCIENCE BEHIND FASTING

Intermittent fasting, commonly abbreviated as IF, is a pattern of eating. Most people eat three meals a day with snacks in between; however, intermittent fasting involves periods of eating with fasting, which are periods of not eating, in between. While most diets talk about *what* you should be eating, intermittent fasting pays more attention to *when* you should be eating. There are multiple different forms of intermittent fasting, including popular methods like

- **16/8 intermittent fasting:** Eating for only 8 hours of the day, fasting for 16.
- **5:2 intermittent fasting:** Complete fasting for two days out of the week.

But how does it work? What is so special about intermittent fasting that allows it to impact weight loss, health, energy, and more? Well, it all boils down to how intermittent fasting impacts your cells and hormones.

First, intermittent fasting impacts human growth hormone, a hormone responsible for our growth, metabolism, and overall health. When you engage in fasting, especially the fasting patterns of intermittent fasting, the body experiences an increase in its levels of human growth hormone. As a result, one can experience fat loss and muscle preservation during a fast, and these benefits are only amplified during more extended fasts. It has also been noted that higher levels of human growth hormone can improve muscle and bone health.

In addition, intermittent fasting plays a role in your insulin levels. Insulin regulates our blood sugar levels, directly controlling how much sugar—or glucose, to be specific—is taken into our cells. When you engage in a fast, especially intermittent fasting, your insulin levels decrease. This means that the body has to use stored fat for energy, burning up fat cells and controlling weight loss, rather than relying on glucose or sugars from food. Such a benefit can also help reduce your risk of type 2 diabetes.

Furthermore, you can experience cellular repair thanks to a strong habit of intermittent fasting. Specifically, intermittent fasting is linked to higher rates of autophagy, a process by which your cells remove or recycle damaged parts. Fasting is actually a trigger for autophagy, meaning that fasting plays a direct role in the repair of cells and removal of parts that are not working. Autophagy is so important because healthy cells can prevent diseases, including neurodegenerative conditions.

Finally, gene expression is impacted by intermittent fasting. There are two proteins, sirtuins and FOXO proteins, that play a role in regulating our gene expression and the function of our cells. Fortunately for us, intermittent fasting can activate these proteins and, therefore, contribute to increased stress resistance and positive gene expression, both resulting in better metabolic health.

To sum that up, the science of intermittent fasting revolves around how intermittent fasting impacts hormones and cellular responses. While everyone experiences somewhat different results from their own intermittent fasting practice, you are likely to encounter several of these benefits—and the benefits to be discussed later—thanks to intermittent fasting.

FASTING: MYTH VS. FACT

Intermittent fasting is a scientific concept, and yet there are dozens of misconceptions that surround intermittent fasting. You might even believe in a few of these misconceptions and not know it! In order to help you truly understand the ins and outs of intermittent fasting, let's break down some of those myths—and replace them with facts—now.

Myth 1: Breakfast Is the Most Important Meal of the Day

Often, we hear that breakfast is the most important meal of the day. Usually, this is with reference to eating a healthy breakfast to set you up for success for the rest of the day. What if I told you that the idea that breakfast is the most important meal of the day is a complete myth?

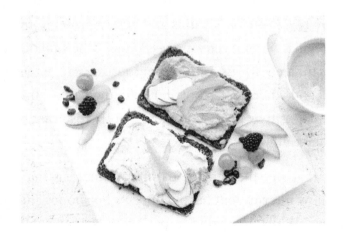

Eating breakfast actually depends on your schedule and preferences. If you wake up hungry or have a fasting window that begins with breakfast, then a nutritious meal can give you a boost of energy and help with your blood sugar levels. Simultaneously, skipping breakfast is perfectly okay if you are not hungry. And besides, there is research that suggests that breaking your fast *later* in the day can have marked health benefits like improving metabolism.

With that being said, breakfast *can* be the most important meal of the day, but it is not inherently. It depends on you and your lifestyle, so do not worry if fasting eliminates breakfast; this is perfectly fine if you are not a breakfast person or sleep late, for instance!

Myth 2: Starvation Mode

Another myth that fasters are frequently confronted with is the idea that fasting puts your body into starvation mode—a state where your body preserves fat for survival rather than burning it. While not eating *can* do this, fasting and starvation are not one and the same. In fact, when it comes to short-term fasting, your metabolism can be boosted rather than shut down (what people commonly believe happens to cause starvation mode). When you fast, the insulin levels in your body lower so that your body eats away at fat rather than glucose. This is the exact reason why proper intermittent fasting does not achieve starvation mode.

Myth 3: Eat Less, More Often

In addition, many people believe that eating less per meal but having more frequent meals is a good weight management strategy. And for some people, it is; it can prevent binge eating, overeating, and other common struggles pertaining to weight gain. However, it is not true that eating less and more frequently *always* leads to weight loss. For a lot of people, this can actually raise glucose levels and result in less weight gain.

Myth 4: Intermittent Fasting = Muscle Loss

Some people believe that intermittent fasting can result in the loss of muscle mass, which is also a myth! As mentioned earlier, intermittent fasting can actually result in muscle retention and growth, not loss. If you are fasting and notice muscle loss, the likely culprit is either a lack of exercise or protein within your diet—which, by the way, can occur to anyone, even those who do not fast!

Myth 5: You Must Fast for 16+ Hours

There are a lot of people who believe that fasting must take a minimum of 16 hours for results to show. This is not true either! Intermittent fasting can be effective even if you fast for just 12 hours. In fact, fasting for different lengths of time can have different benefits across the board, which means that it is vital to understand fasting times and their benefits individually as opposed to making blanket assumptions.

There are dozens of other myths surrounding intermittent fasting, but you'll certainly find those to be dispelled as we continue our journey together. What rings true is that many aspects of what you know about intermittent fasting could be a myth; as you read, remain curious and do not be afraid to learn something new!

FASTING TYPES, EXPLAINED

Did you know that there are more than a half dozen types of intermittent fasting? It's true! And while some are more popular than others, each form of fasting has distinct characteristics and benefits. You can even combine more than one type of intermittent fasting for results, depending on what you start with. This section explains to you the six most popular types of intermittent fasting.

The first type of fasting to understand is 14-hour fasting, sometimes called 14/10 fasting. This method of fasting involves a 14-hour fasting window, followed by a 10-hour eating window. Returning to the myth that only 16+ hour fasts are effective, 14-hour fasting can be equally as effective as a 16-hour fast in many regards—if you play your cards right, that is. One of the major benefits of 14/10 fasting is the fact that the fasting window is slightly shorter than 16/8 fasting, accommodating social scenarios and diverse needs when it comes to fasting. At the same time, depending on your goals, 16-hour fasting might be slightly more effective.

Sixteen-hour fasting, also called 16/8 fasting, is a method of fasting where you have a feeding window of eight hours a day. For most people, 16/8 fasting works well; it helps achieve myriad benefits while also fitting into the day naturally, allowing for one to two meals a day and even social eating, such as dinner with a friend. When considering intermittent fasting, 16/8 fasting is perhaps the most popular form of fasting. However, do not be fooled—16/8 fasting is not the only beneficial form of fasting!

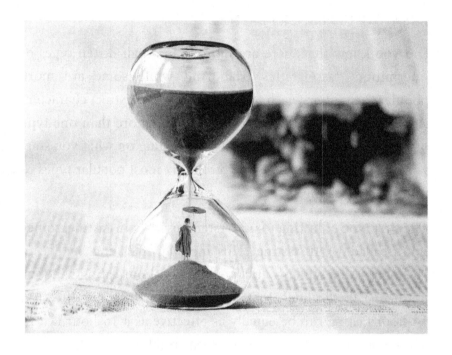

There is also 5:2 fasting. 5:2 fasting involves fasting for two days out of the week, then eating normally for the remaining five. This can be done in two different ways. On the one hand, you can fast for two 24-hour periods throughout the week nonconsecutively; on the other, you have the option of fasting for two consecutive days. Most people opt for the former option, as the latter can be a lot for those new to intermittent fasting. Furthermore, fasting for 48 hours consecutively can be dangerous without the proper preparation, so be careful if this is the option you choose!

Some people choose a fasting method called alternate-day fasting for their needs. During alternate-day fasting, every other day is a fast day. For example, if you fast on Monday, then you'll eat normally on Tuesday and fast again on Wednesday. Alternate-day fasting is beneficial because it is incredibly versatile; on fasting days, for instance, you can do a 16/8 fast, a 24-hour fast, or some other variation of fasting to fit your needs. This balances a fasting lifestyle with one where you maintain the benefits of fasting as well.

And lastly, we cannot forget the warrior diet. The warrior diet is a fasting cycle where you have a 20-hour fasting window followed by a four-hour feeding window. This is a cycle that repeats every single day, which might seem extreme at first, but it is actually very effective. The benefits mentioned earlier, including improved fat burning, muscle build, bone health, and more, can all be obtained from a 20-hour fast cycle. The warrior diet is one of the most effective fasting cycles, but do not feel pressured to jump right into it; most people build up from smaller fasting windows!

GENERAL BENEFITS OF INTERMITTENT FASTING

We've covered a couple of the benefits associated with intermittent fasting, but in order to truly appreciate intermittent fasting for what it is, we have to dive into the benefits. Just a few of the benefits that you can appreciate as a result of intermittent fasting include

- **Decreased brain fog.** A lot of the foods that we eat, especially over-processed foods or foods full of chemicals, can create brain fog, making it hard to focus or concentrate. Intermittent fasting can reduce the signs of brain fog by improving digestion and our ability to process foods.
- **Lower risk for diabetes.** As mentioned earlier, fasting encourages the body to eat away at fat rather than glucose. This lowers insulin levels and, consequently, your risk of diabetes.
- **Protection for the heart.** Some research has indicated that fasting can lower your risk of heart-related ailments. This is due to weight loss, how intermittent fasting impacts your hormones, and more.
- **Reduced inflammation.** Inflammation occurs due to many reasons, including the food we eat. When you fast, however, it gives your body time to clear out toxins and other impacts of the food that you eat, reducing inflammation in the process.
- **Less age-related diseases.** Better nutrition is associated with less age-related diseases, and fasting certainly plays a role. Through the aforementioned hormonal impacts of fasting, your risk of age-related diseases can be lessened.
- **Higher quality sleep.** Fasting can improve your quality of sleep! It helps regulate your circadian rhythms and other bodily processes responsible for sleep, which can make it easier for you to sleep more consistently and with higher quality.

- **Increased cell repair.** As mentioned earlier in the chapter, IF speeds up and facilitates bodily processes that make cell repair easier. This cell repair aids in the prevention of illness and disease.
- **Lower cholesterol/blood pressure.** Intermittent fasting can also help reduce cholesterol and blood pressure.

And that's just the start; we also need to discuss the benefits specific to women over 50—giving you a solid idea of why intermittent fasting is perfect for you!

IF AND WOMEN IN THEIR 50S

In addition to the general benefits mentioned above, there are also specific benefits that intermittent fasting accomplishes for women in their 50s and older. These specific benefits are probably what you are looking for, as you want to tailor intermittent fasting to your needs. Do not worry—I've got you covered when it comes to the benefits of intermittent fasting for women just like you. And remember, each of these benefits will be enumerated in the coming chapter, so if you have more questions by the end of this section, keep on reading.

First, intermittent fasting results in notable weight loss, especially for those over 50 who try it. Hormonal changes, body composition shifts, and changes to metabolism from aging, menopause, and more can make weight retention and even weight gain one of your biggest problems. Fortunately, intermittent fasting can not only eliminate many of the symptoms of these ailments, but it can also drive weight loss.

Furthermore, intermittent fasting has the power to improve metabolic health, something a lot of women struggle with later in life. Because fasting encourages the body to eat away at existing fat stores, it can ramp up your metabolism. This means that the food you eat is absorbed as nutrients, while fat is eaten up for energy. As a result, weight loss is at an all-time high while metabolic health improves as well.

Truly, that's just a fraction of the benefits that can be experienced thanks to intermittent fasting. As we move into Chapter 2, you are sure to find numerous other benefits—alongside an in-depth exploration of the changes you are going to experience—that help you understand your journey more completely.

SUMMARY BOX

The benefits of intermittent fasting include

- Improved fat burning, muscle protection, and bone health.
- Lowered insulin levels for better fat burning and lower risk of diabetes.
- Higher rate of cellular repair and, therefore, reduced risk of certain diseases.
- Better metabolic health through gene expression and stress resistance.
- Decreased brain fog and increased focus.
- Lower cholesterol, inflammation, and blood pressure.
- Marked benefits for women over 50.

These are just some of them; there are many more.

As you can see, intermittent fasting is a beneficial practice with much to be gained, especially for women over 50! Between weight loss, muscle preservation, and more, you can't go wrong by finding the intermittent fasting technique that works for you. As we move into the next chapter, we will endeavor to understand the changes that you're experiencing or will experience in your 50s. This is an important aspect of laying the foundation for developing an intermittent fasting plan, so you definitely don't want to miss this.

PART II

AGING AND NUTRITION

2

THE AGE OF CHANGE— HORMONES AND HEALTH POST- 50

> *Women, our bodies change drastically in comparison to men. We're going through menopause. We've got a lot going on, and I don't think we've done enough to understand what aging means for women's bodies: What are we supposed to look like? How are we supposed to feel? We're not talking about that enough.*
>
> — MICHELLE OBAMA

Aging is a drastically different experience for women than it is for men. One of the biggest changes that you will experience is menopause, a major shift in hormones and the trajectory of your body from here on out. It can be frightening to not know what your body is up to and how to handle it, and that's just the start of the battle. In this chapter, you will find a roadmap to the changes that you are experiencing. This includes a look at hormonal and bodily shifts, as well as how intermittent fasting plays a role.

OVERALL HORMONAL CHANGES

Nearing and after the age of 50, there are countless hormonal changes that you, as a woman, can expect to experience. And while everyone perceives and navigates these changes differently, understanding them in the first place is key when it comes to successfully managing symptoms and living your best life. So, what hormonal changes can you expect to experience after 50 years old?

Aging brings about changes to the body, particularly the endocrine system. The endocrine system is responsible for producing and secreting hormones, which contribute to the regulation of biological processes. Some hormones that shift with age include

- **Estrogen:** During perimenopause and menopause especially, the female body begins to produce less estrogen. As a result, the body can struggle with tasks like maintaining bone density, regulating the menstrual cycle, and supporting reproductive health—causing a plethora of other issues on its own.
- **Prolactin:** Prolactin is responsible for helping with breastfeeding. Specifically, during pregnancy, prolactin levels increase so that one can breastfeed. However, during later stages in life, prolactin levels decrease drastically.

- **Aldosterone:** Aldosterone is responsible for managing our fluid and electrolyte levels. In other words, this is the hormone responsible for balancing salt and water within our bodies. While age does not necessarily impact aldosterone as it does other hormones, you may experience changes in your sensitivity to aldosterone, thus resulting in blood pressure shifts.
- **Calcitonin:** Specifically responsible for bone health and the calcium levels in your blood, age can impact calcitonin production and, therefore, contribute to bone loss.
- **Human growth hormone:** Responsible for tissue repair and growth, metabolism, and the health of bones and muscles, growth hormone can decline with age and impact the body in numerous ways.

Despite all of these changes, the good news is that intermittent fasting can have myriad positive impacts on such hormonal changes. For example, we talked about how intermittent fasting can impact insulin sensitivity in Chapter 1. This impact can actually tie into hormone regulation, especially for those experiencing the aftereffects of menopause. In addition, fasting has been linked to increased secretion of human growth hormone, which can counteract some of the negative impacts of menopause as well.

MENOPAUSE AND METABOLISM

Understanding menopause is good, but let's make our knowledge *great*. We have to dig into the impacts of menopause and what is changing during menopause for true understanding!

Menopause is a natural bodily process that occurs in females during the end of their reproductive years. It's the time when you—usually—stop having a period, your body changes, and you experience big shifts in life as a result. Officially, menopause is considered to be the period after the absence of a period for 12 months in a row. Usually, women experience menopause between their late 40s and early 50s, but some people as young as 20 can experience menopause.

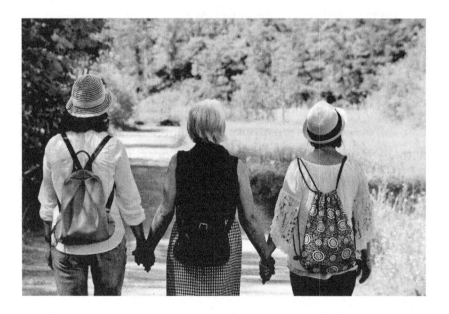

There are countless changes occurring to the body during menopause. Just to name a few, you may experience changes in

- **Hormones:** As mentioned, the production of various hormones fluctuates during menopause, resulting in many of the symptoms you hear about pertaining to menopause.
- **Periods:** Your periods, formerly known as menstrual cycles, will begin to become lighter, heavier, or more irregular. This is perfectly normal when it comes to menopause.
- **Hot flashes:** You might experience sudden and intense feelings of warmth, including more outward signs like sweating. Often, hot flashes can be uncomfortable.
- **Bladder control:** Menopause can cause your pelvic muscles to weaken, resulting in incontinence or urinary urgency.
- **Sleep:** Sleep disturbances are not uncommon for those experiencing menopause. Such disturbances include insomnia and night sweats and can relate to hormonal fluctuations.
- **Vaginal health and sexuality:** Changes in sexual health can arise from vaginal dryness and discomfort typical of menopause.
- **Mood:** You may experience mood swings, irritability, and vulnerability to stress as well.

Beyond that, menopause has a significant impact on your metabolism. Estrogen is impacted during menopause, and the decline in muscle mass that results can contribute to a slower metabolism. Furthermore, hormonal shifts can lead to higher levels of fat retention and can contribute specifically to weight gain. You do not have to feel hopeless about these concerns, however; intermittent fasting has marked benefits not just for your metabolism, but for all of the symptoms of menopause as well!

Intermittent fasting can improve metabolic rate, potentially canceling out some of the hormonal impacts on metabolism due to menopause. This is primarily due to the fact that IF has the power to improve our insulin sensitivity. As a result, not only will you achieve higher hormone regulation during an otherwise tumultuous time, but your weight will be more manageable as well. Moreover, intermittent fasting can contribute to lessening menopause-related inflammation and lowering pain, too!

So, while menopause involves significant changes to your body and impacts various aspects of your health, intermittent fasting can be the secret to not only regaining control over your life but also optimizing your health in a way you've not yet experienced. How exciting is that?

DIGGING INTO SYMPTOMS

In order to really harness the powers of intermittent fasting, I want to spend some time digging into the symptoms of menopause. Specifically, I want to talk about what brings about some of the most treacherous impacts of menopause, as well as how intermittent fasting can be particularly helpful in negating these impacts—or at least making them a little easier to manage. Without further ado, let's delve into menopause symptoms with some more nuance.

Hot Flashes and Night Sweats

First up, we have hot flashes and night sweats. Hot flashes, as discussed earlier, are sudden and intense feelings of heat. Usually, you are going to feel a hot flash in the upper body areas, including the face and neck. This is one of the most common symptoms of menopause, and it can occur at any time of the day or night. We are not sure exactly why hot flashes happen, but the culprit is believed to be how changes in estrogen impact the hypothalamus—the part of the brain responsible for regulating our temperature. Due to hormonal changes, the brain can misperceive the temperature of the body. Common symptoms of a hot flash include sudden feelings of warmth, rapid heartbeat, flushed skin, and sweating followed by a chill.

Night sweats are a bit different. Night sweats involve episodes of sweating during sleep. Usually, night sweats will be triggered by a hot flash. Many women abhor night sweats, as they can wake you up, cause discomfort, and overall contribute to fatigue. Declining estrogen levels are responsible for night sweats, as the decline impacts your body's ability to regulate temperature. Common symptoms of night sweats include intense sweating at night, drenched bedsheets and sleepwear, disturbed sleeping patterns, and anxiety or discomfort.

Intermittent fasting can aid in the reduction of many of these symptoms. For example, the improved insulin sensitivity that you gain from intermittent fasting can lower the fluctuations that you experience when it comes to your blood sugar. This can help prevent hot flashes. In addition, IF helps with

- **Inflammation:** Intermittent fasting can help reduce inflammation throughout the body. This is because fasting gives your body time to process and remove toxins, among other things. Many people are not aware that inflammation can make menopausal symptoms worse, but this little-known fact is why fasting is so good for menopausal symptoms. Because inflammation can exacerbate hot flashes and night sweats in particular, fasting intermittently can remedy such symptoms.

- **Hormones:** As mentioned earlier, menopause impacts several hormones that are responsible for many of our physiological functions. Specifically, menopause can impact our ability to perceive and respond to temperature, our digestion, and more. When it comes to hormonal balance, IF is a superhero; intermittent fasting can influence hormonal balance for hormones that are used by the hypothalamus. As a result, hot flashes can be reduced and temperature regulation improved.

- **Weight:** Finally, intermittent fasting can help improve weight management. It might not be immediately clear how this would reduce hot flashes or night sweats; however, hot flashes, night sweats, and other symptoms of menopause can be reduced through weight management and maintaining a healthy weight.

As you can see, IF has the power to help with hot flashes and night sweats specifically, and that's just one example of how intermittent fasting can benefit those experiencing the symptoms of menopause.

Mood Swings

In addition to hot flashes and night sweats, mood swings are a common side effect of menopause. Many women experience mood swings, which impact not only themselves but those around them. It can be uncomfortable and even somewhat embarrassing to experience mood swings, and that's only half of it if you are unsure of what's going on.

In order to foster an enhanced understanding of mood swings, let's touch on five common reasons that you may experience mood swings as a result of menopause:

1. **Hormonal fluctuations:** Hormonal fluctuations, specifically fluctuations in estrogen and progesterone, can result in mood swings. This is because such hormonal changes impact our neurotransmitters—chemical messengers that communicate between each part of the brain. When neurotransmitters like serotonin and norepinephrine are impacted by hormonal changes, it can be easy to wax and wane between positive and negative emotions rapidly.
2. **Impact on stress response:** Menopause and the resultant effects can also influence the ways in which you respond to stress. Estrogen is particularly influential when it comes to the stress response system; thus, the reduced estrogen levels faced during

menopause can make you more sensitive to stressors. And we all know that heightened levels of stress can contribute to irritability, frustration, and anxiety.

3. **Sleep disruptions:** Night sweats and other sleep disturbances as a result of menopause can mean that you navigate each day tired, exhausted, and generally in a bad mood. As anyone who experiences sleep disturbances knows, not getting enough sleep or getting poor quality sleep can leave you irritable and annoyed throughout the day. Snappiness is not uncommon, either.

4. **Physical symptoms:** Menopause is accompanied by a lot of physical changes. Besides physical symptoms like hot flashes, the slowed metabolic experiences that you have can result in weight gain. And beyond that, your body composition can change drastically during menopause as well. All of this can contribute to concerns about your body image and impact your emotional well-being, which can make it easy for emotions to waver drastically throughout the day.

5. **Life transitions:** Menopause is a transitional period in more ways than one. Not only are your body and life changing in unprecedented ways, but the changes that you are experiencing during menopause can coincide with other major life changes. Children leaving home, career transitions, and more can all lead to inconsistent moods.

Fortunately, intermittent fasting can help manage ever-changing moods with ease. Beyond what I've already mentioned regarding insulin and hormones, IF is immensely beneficial. Intermittent fasting can have neurological benefits, benefiting the health of your brain and mood regulation. Further, a healthy and managed weight can lead to more pleasant moods, and mindfulness associated with IF is great for mood and emotional resilience as well.

At the same time, it would be dishonest to say that IF is without flaw when it comes to mood swings; in some cases, IF can *cause* mood swings. However, these are usually temporary and boil down to a few explainable causes, such as the initial adaptation period from changing your diet. This will be elaborated upon in Chapter 7, so do not worry about this for now.

Sleeping Patterns

It's no surprise that many women experience sleep issues during their menopausal phase. There is so much going on, and naturally, those changes and struggles contribute to issues with sleep. In general, there are five main ways that menopause contributes to poor sleeping patterns and disturbances:

1. **Hormonal fluctuations:** The decline of estrogen and other hormones as a result of menopause can result in the dysfunction and dysregulation of neurotransmitters, including melatonin. As you may know, melatonin is directly responsible and crucial for our sleep-wake cycles. Without melatonin, we may not sleep long enough or have good quality sleep, for example. Menopause directly impacts your melatonin production.

2. **Night sweats:** Understandably so, it can be immensely difficult to sleep when experiencing hot flashes or night sweats, either separately or together. Feeling like your bedroom is scorching and sleeping in a puddle of sweat isn't exactly conducive to restful sleep. Because of this, you might experience disrupted sleeping patterns that leave you feeling groggy or exhausted the next day.

3. **Sleep disorders:** Sleep disorders like insomnia, sleep apnea, and more tend to increase with age. This means that as you get older, your chances of experiencing a sleep disorder are higher. Such sleep disorders are only exacerbated thanks to menopause and related changes.

4. **Psychological factors:** Hormonal changes, lifestyle changes, and other major changes in life can result in stress and anxiety. Heightened psychological factors—especially those as a result of menopause—may contribute to reduced sleep quality.

5. **Circadian rhythm changes:** With age comes the natural change of circadian rhythms—the cycles in our body that help us understand when to wake up and go to sleep. Of course, changing circadian rhythm cycles will throw off your ability to get a restful night's sleep.

While there are significant factors that can contribute to poor sleep during menopause, intermittent fasting has been linked to improved sleep as well. Between improved hormonal balance and IF's ability to improve circadian rhythm alignment, reduce inflammation, and improve brain health, you are in good hands when it comes to improving your sleep through intermittent fasting.

Changes in Heart Health

Heart health and the detrimental impact of menopause on heart health can be one of the more frightening and disparaging impacts of hitting such an age. In addition, there are special considerations that need to be made regarding heart health and fasting, so it is important that you read through this section carefully.

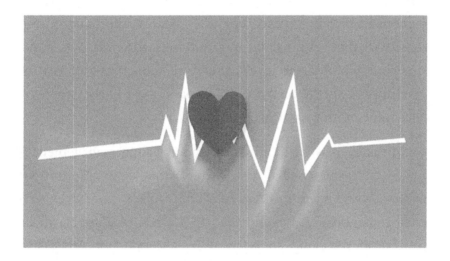

There are various changes to heart health that you can experience as you age. Estrogen is a powerhouse when it comes to protecting the heart, including the promotion of healthy blood vessels and reduced inflammation. However, because estrogen levels decline during menopause, it is possible that you will experience cardiovascular health issues. Moreover, aging results in the hardening of arteries, which can land you with higher blood pressure and an increased risk of heart attack.

Interestingly enough, women are also more susceptible to something called "broken heart" syndrome, more formerly known as takotsubo cardiomyopathy. It's a real condition that results from the loss of a loved one. It pertains specifically to the emotional distress that accompanies loss and can mimic the symptoms of a heart attack.

At the same time, intermittent fasting can play a role in improving your heart health and protecting against menopausal heart impacts. For example, the improved insulin sensitivity that results from intermittent fasting can help regulate your blood sugar levels, therefore reducing your risk of insulin resistance. Because of this, you are less likely to experience issues with your heart.

Additionally, it is well known that poor weight management is linked to cardiovascular risk factors; thanks to intermittent fasting, however, this is less of a concern for women experiencing menopause. Beyond that, IF stimulates autophagy, the process of repairing damaged cells. Through this process of maintaining cell integrity, your heart can maintain its health.

If you experience existing heart conditions or are at risk of developing one, as indicated by family history or diagnosis, you'll want to consider a few things before jumping right into intermittent fasting. Understand first that IF can impact everyone differently, which is especially the case when you are experiencing menopause and fasting.

Individual variability is important to consider, which means you should keep in mind factors like the state of your overall health, any existing health or heart conditions that you have, and any genetic predispositions that might come into play. If any of these aspects fit you, make sure to talk with your doctor or primary care physician before starting to IF regularly.

Inflammation

Inflammation and aging are something else that you need to consider when it comes to understanding your body's changes and your IF journey. Inflammation is a common symptom that women in later stages of life experience. Particularly, chronic and low-grade inflammation is common among older women. Age-related inflammation is also associated with age-related diseases, including heart disease, diabetes, and neurodegenerative conditions. Beyond that, inflammation can result in joint pain, hot flashes, and other uncomfortable symptoms.

Something that plays a particular role in age-related inflammation in various parts of the body is macrophages. Macrophages are immune cells that have a vital role in how our immune system responds to various stimuli. As you age, your macrophages can become dysregulated, resulting in increased inflammation. This is because your body can view benign activity or any new input as a threat, causing inflammation to "fight" it rather than parsing through the data. Simultaneously, during aging, cells can enter a state referred to as *senescence*. This means that cells stop dividing to produce new cells but remain metabolically active. These cells can cause inflammation and attract macrophages, making the inflammation even worse —and, at times, chronic.

Intermittent fasting can be a particularly excellent way to reduce inflammation. By now, you are probably well acquainted with how intermittent fasting can stimulate autophagy. This allows the body to clean up and reduce the burden of senescent cells, therefore decreasing inflammation. Moreover, IF can have direct anti-inflammatory effects all on its own by lowering the levels of inflammatory markers within the bloodstream. Between this, regulating immune cells, improving insulin sensitivity, and reducing oxidative stress that contributes to inflammation, IF is a golden tactic for lowering your inflammation overall.

Bone and Muscle Health

The last main change that we have to discuss is bone and muscle health. Changes in your bone and muscle density are caused by hormonal shifts primarily, and there are a few different conditions from which you might suffer that negatively impact the bones and muscles:

- **Osteoporosis:** Characterized by weakened and porous bones, osteoporosis can increase your risk of fracturing a bone. Aging is a significant risk factor when it comes to developing osteoporosis, and your chances of developing the condition increase after menopause.
- **Osteoarthritis:** A degenerative joint disease resulting from the breakdown of cartilage in the joints, with aging as the primary risk factor due to age-related wear and tear.

- **Rheumatoid arthritis:** An autoimmune disease causing inflammation in the joints. It can occur at any age, but the chances of development do increase with age.

IF can be stellar for alleviating the symptoms of bone and muscle health. IF increases human growth hormone, for instance, which enables your body to strengthen bones and muscles as opposed to allowing them to degrade. Furthermore, the hormonal balance associated with intermittent fasting can allow you to achieve more retention of bone and muscle mass, improving your health overall.

As you can see, there are a lot of health conditions associated with aging and menopause that can be quite difficult to manage. But when you have intermittent fasting by your side, healing and growth are more accessible than ever.

SUMMARY BOX

Some of the changes you may be experiencing during and after the age of 50 include

- Hormonal changes to estrogen, prolactin, aldosterone, calcitonin, and human growth hormone.
- Menopausal symptoms include but are not limited to changes in bone or muscle density, hot flashes, sleep concerns, metabolic shifts, and more.
- Damage to the health of the heart, increased inflammation, and loss of bone or muscle mass.

There are a lot of changes that accompany menopause, and some of them can be quite scary. However, you do not have to feel victimless to some of the more harrowing symptoms, including symptoms that slowly deteriorate your body from the inside out. Instead, let's turn to IF for the solution—a simple practice that can help you achieve big results. In the next chapter, we're going to focus on the nutrient needs of aging women and how understanding these nutrient needs can impact your fasting journey. A lot of people worry about not getting enough nutrients while fasting, so Chapter 3 is your key to preventing this!

3

NOURISHMENT IN YOUR 50S— MEETING YOUR NUTRITIONAL MILESTONES

 To eat is a necessity, but to eat intelligently is an art.

— FRANÇOIS DE ROCHEFOUCAULD

Anyone can eat. We eat every day—well, most of us do. Eating is one of the most important facets of life because it is through food that we sustain ourselves. With that being said, one can truly consider eating with tact and intelligence to be a form of art! Not everyone understands the intricate balance between nutrition, feeding windows, and caring for the body. One of the many things that this book is going to help you uncover is how exactly you can meet your nutritional milestones through the art of intelligent eating.

BENEFITS OF GOOD NUTRITION

We often hear that it's important to have good nutrition, but what is good nutrition in the first place? Depending on who you ask, you're going to get varying definitions; some people might argue that good nutrition involves simply eating enough fruits and vegetables, while others argue that nutrition depends entirely on the person. Neither is wrong, but neither is completely correct, either.

Good nutrition involves a blend of three aspects: micronutrients, macronutrients, and hydration. These three factors of nutrition must all be in balance in order for one to say that they have "good" nutrition. Now, this does have an element of individualization; everyone needs different levels of these nutrients —which we will talk about in the coming sections—in order to be in good health. Simultaneously, eating enough fruits and vegetables matters, but they're not the only thing that does matter when it comes to good nutrition.

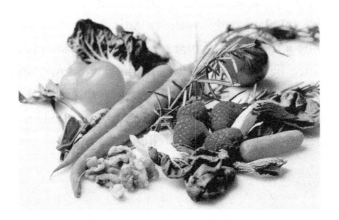

In the next several sections, you'll come to understand exactly what makes up good nutrition. However, let's spend some time focusing on just a few of the benefits that women 50 and older can experience from good nutrition, hopefully motivating you to care about nutrition as a vital component of your IF journey:

- **Reduced risk of some diseases:** This includes heart disease, diabetes, stroke, some cancers, and osteoporosis. When you eat enough and get all of the right nutrients, you have the ability to fight off disease. This is because your body is equipped to fight off disease through nutrition, which is important—it is even harder to have good nutrition at 50 than it is at 15.
- **Reduces high blood pressure:** Certain foods are associated with reduced levels of blood pressure, which is certainly a good thing considering many women over 50 suffer from high blood pressure. And in turn, this lowered blood pressure can help you live longer and healthier!
- **Lowers high cholesterol:** Cholesterol can build up in the heart and arteries due to both age and poor nutrition. However, when you eat right, your cholesterol levels can lower—reducing your risk of heart attack and stroke as a result.
- **Improves your well-being:** Generally speaking, well-being is improved through good nutrition. Both mental and physical well-being can be boosted through eating enough of the right things, and that isn't even to mention how the right foods can alleviate menopause symptoms and signs of aging.

- **Improves your ability to fight off illness:** Nutrition is the main way to empower your immune system to fight off illness. Many people recommend consuming lots of vitamin C to fend off a cold, which can certainly help; at the same time, all nutrients are valuable for maintaining health and resilience against illness.
- **Improves your ability to recover from illness or injury:** Good nutrition flows to every part of the body, including the bones and muscles. This can help your body overcome external and internal injuries and illnesses alike.
- **Increases your energy level:** Additionally, eating enough of the right nutrients can be the secret to overcoming grogginess and low energy, especially the drained energy levels associated with menopause and aging.

Truly, nutrition is a gateway into strong and powerful health that truly allows you to live your best life. And even when you're fasting, you can still care about nutrition for your feeding windows. In order to help you understand specific aspects of nutrition, let's take a look at one of the three components of strong nutrition—micronutrients.

THE MICRONUTRIENT POWERHOUSE

The prefix "micro" means "small," which is exactly what micronutrients are—small nutrients that stack for big benefits! More specifically, micronutrients are nutrients that the body needs in smaller amounts compared to other nutrients. These nutrients are vital for the body, as they power our physiological functions (such as nerve function, cell production, and more). Vitamins and minerals are common micronutrients, and they are needed in a much smaller quality than macronutrients.

Vitamin B12

When it comes to micronutrients that are particularly important for women over 50, there are seven we can consider. The first micronutrient that we're going to talk about is vitamin B12. Vitamin B12 is the micronutrient specifically responsible for nerve function, as well as the production of red blood cells. This means that you need enough vitamin B12 for healthy nerves, blood functioning, and overall well-being. You need about 2.4 micrograms of vitamin B12 a day, which might sound like very little, but some people struggle to obtain even that! Luckily, vitamin B12 can be found in a variety of easily accessible foods, like meat, fish, dairy, and fortified foods.

Vitamin B6

Then, there is vitamin B6. Vitamin B6 may be another B vitamin, but it serves an idiosyncratic purpose when it comes to physical health—meaning that just because you have enough B12 doesn't mean you have enough B6, and vice versa. Vitamin B6 is responsible for various functions of its own, which can include functions like brain development and the function of neurotransmitters. In other words, vitamin B6 empowers the brain to communicate between different components of itself, and then *act* on those communications intelligently. It is recommended that you consume between 1.5 and 2 micrograms of vitamin B6 a day, and you can source vitamin B6 from food sources like chicken, turkey, fish, potatoes, and bananas.

Magnesium

Magnesium is another important micronutrient for everyone to have, but that's doubly the case for women over 50. You might know that magnesium is one of the valuable nutrients for alleviating period cramps and other symptoms, but it can also help with menopause symptoms. Beyond that, magnesium serves the purpose of helping with muscle and nerve function, improving bone health, and maximizing energy production. Magnesium is crucial and carries out so many different functions, which is why many people need up to or just over 320 per day. Magnesium is found in foods like leafy green vegetables, nuts, seeds, whole grains, and legumes.

Omega-3 Fatty Acids

Omega-3 fatty acids are another micronutrient that is important for your well-being. Omega-3s aren't necessarily vitamins, but they are valuable to health, considering the fact that they influence heart health and brain function. Beyond that, they can also reduce inflammation. There are two main forms of omega-3 fatty acids that you should consume, EPA and DHA, and you need between 250 and 500 milligrams of the two *combined*. There are many supplements and natural sources from which you can derive omega-3s, including fatty fish, chia and flax seeds, and walnuts.

Vitamin D

Another important micronutrient to consider is vitamin D. You might know vitamin D as the vitamin that you get from spending time in the sunlight, which is true; however, there are several other reasons that you need vitamin D. For example, vitamin D is essential for the absorption of calcium, which contributes to your overall bone health. Moreover, vitamin D is crucial to a properly functioning immune system. It is recommended that you get 600 to 800 international units (IU) of vitamin D per day, which can be more aptly described as 10–30 minutes of strong sunlight exposure several times a week. You can also obtain vitamin D through fatty fish and fortified dairy products.

Calcium

Calcium is important, too. Many people think of calcium as the milk vitamin, which certainly is one good source of it. You can also get calcium through leafy greens and fortified, plant-based milk if you don't drink cow's milk. Women over 50 should consume about 1,200 milligrams of calcium per day. This high number is due to the fact that calcium is necessary for bone health, muscle function, and nerves—all aspects that women over 50 may struggle with when it comes to health.

Potassium

Finally, we have potassium. Potassium is good for the health of the heart and muscles, and it contributes significantly to the balance of fluids within the body as well. You should consume around 2,600 to 3,400 milligrams of potassium per day, which isn't much when you consider the diverse sources from which it comes—like bananas, oranges, potatoes, tomatoes, and leafy green vegetables.

With that being said, it's important to achieve a diverse set of micronutrient inclusions in your diet every single day. But micronutrients are far from all that matters!

BALANCING MACRONUTRIENTS

In addition to micronutrients, your body needs various macronutrients to survive and sustain various functions. Macronutrients are required in larger quantities, at least compared to the micronutrients we mentioned in the last section. Macronutrients provide energy and support different physiological functions within the body. There are three primary macronutrients to be mindful of as a woman over 40.

Carbohydrates

The first macronutrient to consider is carbohydrates. A lot of people think of carbohydrates and associate them with bread, and then come to the conclusion that carbohydrates must be bad for you because bread is bad for you. This flawed line of thinking is riddled with misconceptions that you have to over-come. Bread isn't bad for you; rather, certain types of bread are bad for you.

Beyond that, carbohydrates don't make you gain weight like crazy or damage your health. In fact, carbohydrates are your body's first and most abundant source of energy, which is more important than ever when you hit 50. Carbohydrates can be found in far more food sources than just bread, including other grains, fruits, vegetables, and legumes like beans.

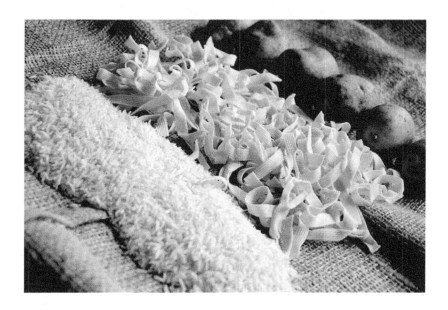

Protein

The second macronutrient to understand is protein. Protein serves many different purposes throughout the body, notably including tissue growth and repair. Protein is vital for the muscles in particular. Beyond that, protein contributes to the production of enzymes and hormones, both essential chemicals in the body. You can absorb protein thanks to the help of numerous food sources, including meat, poultry, fish, certain dairy products, and plant-based sources of protein.

Protein is perhaps the most important macronutrient for women over 50 to pay attention to. Your intake of other macronutrients is important, but protein intake matters a great deal for a few special reasons:

- **Muscle maintenance:** Protein is the most important macronutrient when it comes to maintaining muscle and even growing muscle through avenues like exercise. Women over 50 are especially prone to muscle loss, which means that protein is the key to avoiding such a painful and life-altering symptom of age.
- **Weight management:** Protein is a superhero when it comes to managing weight, even for those to whom weight has been particularly troubling. The reason that protein can be particularly helpful is that it's filling; rather than filling up on non-nutritious, calorically dense foods, filling up on protein can keep weight management troubles at bay.
- **Bone health:** Protein is also a vital component of ensuring that bones remain strong and resilient against damage. Because bone health is such a significant issue for women over 50, protein can make a crucial addition to the diet so that you can maintain strong, healthy bones.
- **Immune support:** Many people think of vitamin C as the only nutrient that you need for immune support, but this is far from true. Protein plays an elemental role in immune support, meaning that if you don't consume enough protein, you could be putting your health, wellness, and recovery at risk.

Therefore, any woman above the age of 50 simply must get enough protein within their diet in order to maintain good health. Your protein intake is vital to ensuring that your body is strong and in working order, inside and out.

Fats

When you hear the word "fat," your brain might be programmed to assume we're talking about something negative; however, this isn't the case at all for dietary fats. In fact, dietary fats are a vital component of balanced nutrition. Specifically, dietary fats are responsible for allowing you to absorb vitamins A, D, E, and K, and they also provide the body with a concentrated source of energy. Beyond that, fats provide structure to our cells and allow them to function. Healthy sources of dietary fat include avocados, nuts, seeds, olive oil, and fatty fish.

Fiber

We haven't mentioned it yet, but fiber is invaluable as well. Fiber is the most important nutrient when it comes to supporting your digestive health. Many women over 50 struggle with constipation, for instance, which fiber can alleviate fast. Moreover, fiber can help control blood sugar levels, which in and of itself is a wonderful way to protect against numerous health issues. Fiber can even aid in weight management, allowing you to feel fuller faster, thus preventing the tendency to overeat. You can find fiber in foods like whole grains, fruits, vegetables, legumes, and nuts.

How Much of Each Do I Need?

Depending on your age, body type, activity level, and more, each person needs a different level of each macronutrient. Generally, it is recommended that you consume 45–65% of your daily calories through carbohydrates, 10–35% through protein, and 20–35% through fats. However, you can calculate your macronutrient needs in just four steps:

1. **Determine your total daily caloric needs.** I recommend asking a dietician what your calorie needs are, but you can also use an online calculator to estimate. Your daily caloric needs are based on factors like age, activity level, and goals.

2. **Allocate macronutrient percentages.** With the recommended percentages above, you can begin to determine grams of each macronutrient based on total daily calories.

3. **Convert percentages to grams.** Using online guides, convert the percentage you need to grams. For instance, if someone eats 2,000 calories daily and wants to consume 30% protein, that's 600 calories in protein since one gram of protein is four calories.

4. **Select balanced food sources.** Based on what you find through your calculations, select balanced food sources that help you meet your goals.

With all of that being said, it's certainly important that you pay attention to your macronutrient intake alongside your micronutrients. Macronutrients are needed in far larger quantities and must be eaten with a particular balance for the most optimal results—especially for women over 50. But there's another facet of nutrition that you may be overlooking, and we have to talk about it.

HYDRATION AND FASTING

Hydration is important for everyone, but when you're not eating due to a fast, hydration is literally a matter of life or death. We get a substantial amount of fluids through foods that contain water, so when you go on a fast, that effectively cuts out a good percentage of your fluid intake. What's more, is that hydration is more important than ever once you hit the age of 50. Now, it's time to take a moment to talk about the importance of hydration and how you can ensure that you're getting enough to drink, whether you're fasting or not!

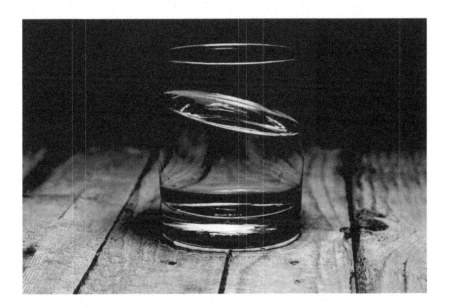

Benefits of Hydration

There are countless benefits that accompany proper hydration, and it's quite unfortunate that so many people lack the knowledge to maintain hydration. For a woman over 50 who is about to begin the journey of intermittent fasting, hydration is of the essence. Just a few of the benefits of good hydration include

- **Helps suppress appetite:** When looking at fasting for the first time, the gripe that many have is with hunger. Fortunately, consistent hydration can suppress hunger both during and outside of IF. This means that water can not only lead to a more successful fast, but it can also improve your weight management.
- **Increases feeling of fullness:** Similarly, water can help the meals that you eat to fill you up more sufficiently. This reduces hunger later during your fasting window, making it easier to stick to the parameters of your diet.
- **Promotes healthy digestion:** Did you know water can improve digestion? Water is necessary to allow digestive processes to flow smoothly. This can help alleviate constipation, improve weight loss, and otherwise contribute to your goals during intermittent fasting.
- **Maintains proper bodily functions:** Without hydration, every part of your body suffers; your brain won't think well, your muscles will cramp, and you will otherwise feel low on energy and in poor health. This can be avoided through proper hydration.
- **Reduces risk of dehydration:** Naturally, remaining hydrated reduces the effects of dehydration, which we will talk about shortly.

As you can see, water is immensely important for your overall well-being. As we continue through this section, you'll unearth everything you need for stellar hydration habits.

Signs of Dehydration

I can't count the number of times someone has told me that they're hydrated while actively experiencing some of the most pertinent signs of dehydration. Because of how prevalent this can be, it's important to know some of the key signs of dehydration:

- **Dark urine:** Urine is, when hydrated, a light yellow, if not almost clear, color. Dark or amber-colored urine is a clear sign of dehydration.
- **Reduced urination:** If you are urinating less often than usual or in a lesser quantity, you are likely suffering from dehydration.
- **Thirst:** Sometimes, things are simple; if you're thirsty, you might be dehydrated. Extreme or excessive thirst can indicate stronger dehydration.
- **Dry skin and/or mouth:** Water is necessary to keep your skin, mouth, and more hydrated. If your skin, mouth, lips, eyes, or other parts of the body feel dryer than usual, you're likely experiencing dehydration.
- **Fatigue and dizziness:** In moderate to severe cases of dehydration, one can become tired or dizzy.
- **Headache:** Many people report experiencing headaches that accompany any degree of dehydration.
- **Sunken eyes:** Sunken eyes can indicate more severe levels of dehydration as well.

- **Confusion:** In some cases, because the brain is unable to function without sufficient water, those who are dehydrated can become confused.
- **Muscle cramps:** Water is vital to the muscles; without it, you are likely to experience pretty bad muscle cramps.

For more severe cases of dehydration, you may need medical attention. Keep in mind that rehydration is done through slow and consistent efforts—not chugging a gallon of water once and leaving it to chance. Remember that dehydration is no joke, and can be life-threatening.

Calculating Hydration Needs

Now that you understand how important water is both in and outside of the scope of a fast, you have to understand how to calculate your particular hydration needs—because the amount of water I need could be vastly different than the amount of water you need. Just like the macronutrients that you need depend on age, activity level, and more, the amount of water that you need depends on various factors. Most specifically, it depends on your weight.

In order to calculate your weight to water needs, you're going to first need to convert your weight to kilograms (which is a more standard unit of measuring weight than pounds). Then, multiply your weight in kilograms by 30–35, which represents milliliters.

From there, divide your value by 29.6, and you will get your ounces of water per day. Here is a sample calculation:

1. Weight = 100 pounds = about 45 kilograms
2. 45 x 35 = 1,575 milliliters of water per day
3. 1,575/29.6 = 53.2 ounces, rounded to 53 for a total of 53 oz of water per day.

If all of that is too much work, you can't go wrong with the 8x8 rule—eight servings of eight ounces of water per day.

Electrolyte Balancing

Electrolytes are different minerals responsible for carrying an electric charge, and they are vital to your body's functioning. They help regulate fluids, support the muscles, transmit nerve signals, and more. Substances like sodium and potassium are just two of the many electrolytes that humans need to survive. Some of the ways that you can balance your electrolytes include

- Stay hydrated by drinking enough water.
- Eat a balanced diet that includes all of the necessary micronutrients *and* macronutrients.
- Be mindful of your sodium intake—not too much, not too little.
- Eat enough potassium, calcium, and magnesium.

It is also important that you have a healthy relationship with sports drinks. While many people simply like Gatorade and other kinds, these are meant for those who exercise to help them replenish their electrolytes. Drinking five Gatorade drinks a day when you lead a sedentary lifestyle isn't good for you. An electrolyte drink once in a while can be immensely helpful in balancing your electrolytes, and they are a wonderful option for those who work out often.

Can You Only Hydrate With Water?

Water is the best source of hydration, and you should treat it as your primary source of hydration. Despite this, you can still hydrate through other sources to meet your hydration needs. Herbal and noncaffeinated teas, milk, and unsweetened and diluted fruit juices can contribute to hydration as well. Fruits and vegetables with a high water content, such as watermelon and cucumber, can also contribute to helping you attain enough water every day. Even something like a soup broth can be a helpful way to sneak in extra hydration.

CREATING YOUR OWN MEAL PLAN

Through learning all of this nutritional information, you might be wondering how you can tailor your nutritional habits to your own needs, effectively creating your very own meal plan. This might seem like a tall order to fill, but the process of creating your own meal plan is actually rather simple:

1. Take a look at your schedule. Before working with recipe planning, it's a good idea to figure out when you will have the time and energy to work with your meal plans. I recommend blocking off specific times that you will dedicate to cooking.

2. Choose some recipes. Based on the recipes below and what you personally enjoy eating, consider some recipes that you would like to include in your meal plan.
3. Put the recipes into your schedule. You have blocked off times and you have recipes. Now, you can plug those recipes into various slots in your schedule so that you know when to make them.
4. Make a grocery list. Write down every ingredient (and quantity) that you will need for all of your recipes. Go through your kitchen and cross out anything you already have. Then, you know what you need to buy.
5. Buy it! Now, you just have to go grocery shopping.
6. Cook, eat, and do it all over! After you have your ingredients, you can cook, enjoy your food, and make meal planning a succinct habit.

FANTASTIC IF RECIPES

Now, it's time to take a look at a few examples of recipes that you can use for your own IF meal-planning journey.

Lemony Salmon Delight

For this recipe, you will need the following ingredients:

- 2 teaspoons of freshly chopped dill
- 1/2 teaspoon of black pepper
- 1/2 teaspoon of salt
- 1/2 teaspoon of garlic powder
- 1 1/2 pounds of salmon filets

- 1/4 cup of firmly packed brown sugar
- 1 chicken bouillon cube, dissolved in 3 tablespoons of water
- 3 tablespoons of oil
- 3 tablespoons of soy sauce
- 4 tablespoons of finely diced green onions
- 1 thinly sliced lemon
- 2 onion slices, separated into rings

Instructions:

1. With your salmon in a shallow glass pan, sprinkle your pepper, salt, dill, and garlic powder over the salmon.
2. Mix the bouillon, oil, soy sauce, green onions, and sugar together in another dish, before pouring this over the salmon.
3. Cover the salmon with cling wrap and chill for an hour, turning once halfway through.
4. Drain and discard the liquid.
5. With your grill on medium heat, put your salmon on the grill to begin cooking it, and then place the lemon and onion on top of the salmon.
6. Cover and cook for 15 minutes or until done.

Cheesy Veggies and Chicken Salad

For this recipe, you will need

- 1 cup of diced, cooked, boneless, skinless chicken breast
- 1/4 cup of finely chopped celery

- 1/4 cup of carrot, shaved into ribbons
- 1/2 cup of baby spinach, roughly chopped
- 2 1/2 tablespoons of fat-free mayonnaise
- 2 tablespoons of nonfat sour cream
- 1/8 teaspoon of dried parsley
- 2 teaspoons of Dijon mustard
- 1/4 cup of shredded reduced-fat sharp cheddar cheese

Instructions:

1. Mix all of the ingredients together, ensuring that the mayonnaise mixture coats all ingredients.
2. Chill in the fridge for 30 minutes or up to overnight.

Cauliflower-Style Popcorn

For this recipe, you will need

- 1 head of cauliflower or an equivalent amount of commercially precut cauliflower
- 4 tablespoons of olive oil
- 1 teaspoon of salt, or more to your liking

Instructions:

1. Preheat the oven to 425 degrees Fahrenheit.
2. Prepare the cauliflower by trimming the head, discarding the core and thick stems, and cutting the florets into pieces approximately the size of ping-pong balls.

3. In a big bowl, whisk together the olive oil and salt. Add the cauliflower pieces to the mixture and toss thoroughly.

4. Spread the cauliflower pieces evenly on the sheet and roast for 1 hour, turning them 3 or 4 times, until a golden brown color develops on most of each piece.

SUMMARY BOX

When considering good nutrition, women over 50 need to pay special attention to the following aspects:

- **Micronutrients:** Minerals and vitamins are needed in smaller quantities to sustain physiological benefits.

- **Macronutrients:** Nutrients are needed in bigger quantities for survival, including carbohydrates and protein.

- **Hydration:** Make sure to drink enough water.

Nourishing your body might seem like a complicated task, but with what you've understood throughout the course of this chapter, it can be far easier to start new nutritional habits that lead to your health today. With that being said, it's time for us to transition into the next part of the book!

PART III

STRATEGIC PLANNING AND INTEGRATION

4

TIMING IS EVERYTHING— CRAFTING YOUR FASTING SCHEDULE

A growing body of research suggests that the timing of the fast is key, and can make intermittent fasting a more realistic, sustainable, and effective approach for weight loss, as well as for diabetes prevention. In this chapter, you're going to uncover the secrets to customizing a fasting window that aligns with your health and lifestyle for optimal safety and effectiveness.

CHOOSING YOUR FASTING WINDOW

Now that you understand the ins and outs of intermittent fasting *and* nutrition, the next step in the process is to pick your fasting window. Your fasting window refers to the duration or times during which you do not eat—effectively meaning that you are fasting. There are many different options when it comes to choosing a fasting window, and those options can even be tailored to your needs and lifestyle. Let's dig in to the best fasting window options for beginners and their benefits!

Daily Fasting Methods

First, we have daily fasting methods. As the name would suggest, daily fasting methods are fasting methods that you engage with every single day. Some people also refer to this as time-restricted eating, because these methods restrict the times of day during which you can eat. As you participate in time-restricted fasting, it is important to emphasize nutrient-rich foods during feeding windows. With that being said, what daily fasting methods can be employed, and which is right for you?

16/8 Intermittent Fasting

The most common method of daily intermittent fasting is 16/8 fasting. During a 16/8 fast, you would fast for 16 hours of the day, using eight hours for your feeding window. For some people, this means skipping breakfast; others snack throughout the feeding window or even just eat one meal a day (commonly called OMAD fasting). Because this method of fasting is flexible, your 16-hour fast can start at any time and end at any time, so long as there are 16 hours of consecutive fasting. For instance, many people fast from 8 p.m. until noon the next day, eating from 12 p.m. until 8 p.m.

16/8 fasting is a popular option for many people because it comes with many benefits. Specifically, 16/8 fasting is wonderful for weight management, as this results in a natural reduction in calorie intake. Many people notice that they lose weight rapidly within the first few weeks of 16/8 fasting.

Moreover, 16/8 fasting is perfect for enhancing insulin sensitivity and thus reducing the risk of type 2 diabetes.

14/10 Intermittent Fasting

14/10 intermittent fasting is another fasting option that you have. During a 14/10 fast, you eat for 10 hours of the day and fast for 14. This is a reduced-intensity version of 16/8 fasting, meaning that it can bring benefits to you that are similar to a 16/8 fast but can be more accommodating to social needs, medical needs, and more. In particular, those who participate in 14/10 fasting on a regular basis say that they experience digestive rest that leads to better digestion, help with weight management, and less stress than 16/8 fasting can accompany. It certainly is the way to go if a gentle approach to fasting is what you seek.

The 5:2 Method

Fasting does not have to be an everyday practice. Some people opt to participate in 5:2 fasting. This method of fasting involves eating normally for five days and fasting for two. Usually, these two fasting days are nonconsecutive. And while the 5:2 fasting method may seem intense, some fasting fans choose to have a low-calorie intake on their two fasting days—usually 500 to 600 calories. This can make 5:2 fasting more accessible without reducing the effectiveness of the method. 5:2 fasting is wonderful for weight loss and heart health!

Fasting Schedule Considerations for Women in Their 50s

Before you commit to a fasting schedule or jump right into fasting, I have to caution you—it is not safe for everyone to fast, and not all fasting schedules are for everyone. Before you commit to a schedule, there are three cardinal rules you must consider:

1. Before you begin any type of intermittent fasting routine, be sure to consider your health status. This includes thinking about any medical conditions you have or medications that you take. For example, some medications must be taken with food. IF isn't safe for all medical conditions without accommodation, so be sure to consult with a doctor if needed.

2. Think about any social commitments, work schedules, or other time-based circumstances that may play a role in your intermittent fasting routine. For instance, people with physically active jobs should be sure to eat beforehand.

3. Make sure that the plan you pick fits into your routine without disrupting your overall lifestyle. You don't have to stop going to brunch with friends; instead, you can readjust your fasting window.

MEDICAL CONSIDERATIONS

In addition to the considerations mentioned at the end of the last section, there are specific medical considerations that you should keep in mind before fasting as well:

- **Hormonal imbalances:** While intermittent fasting can be beneficial for hormonal imbalances, existing hormonal imbalances can also pose an issue for new fasters. Hormonal changes due to aging—and menopause in particular—can influence activity level, energy level, weight distribution, and more. Fasting can make these changes worse if not done with careful consideration.

- **Immune deficiencies:** Immune deficiencies can make fasting somewhat risky. The body can interpret such a massive change as sudden dips in calories or changes in feeding windows as a reason to attack the body to try and stop changes. If you have immune deficiencies or disorders, consult with a doctor before committing to fasting.

- **Medications that suppress the immune system:** Similar to the last point, medication that suppresses the immune system can play a role in whether fasting is right for you. In some cases, fasting can prevent your medication from working in the first place.

- **Eating disorders:** If you have or have had an eating disorder, fasting may not be for you. Fasting can increase the likelihood of recurring eating disorders. Beyond that, if you are prone to eating disorders or have a family history, you might benefit from less intense fasts or consulting with a doctor and a psychiatrist first.

- **Insulin/diabetes:** Because fasting can impact insulin levels significantly, those with diabetes or who take insulin should always consult with a doctor prior to beginning a fast or opting for a particular fasting schedule.

- **Seizure disorders:** Fasting can impact one's likelihood of seizures if they have a seizure disorder or take seizure-related medication.
- **Underweight:** Those who are underweight need to manage fasting carefully, as fasting can make their already low weight even lower.

If you have one of the above conditions, this is not to say that fasting is completely out of the equation; rather, this just means that you may need special accommodations or adjustments for your fasting schedule, which is totally normal. You'll learn how to personalize your fasting schedule later in this chapter!

Impacts of Fasting on Women Over 50

Much like different health conditions can impact fasting, fasting can impact the development of health conditions. While fasting is not going to give you a life-threatening disease or anything of that caliber, it is important to be mindful of the fact that fasting can have side effects—and some of these side effects can be quite alarming. When considering fasting, some impacts you might want to think about include

- **Hypoglycemia (low blood sugar):** Fasting can lead to low blood sugar, because when you are fasting, you are not getting any sugar. Depending on the person, the effects of low blood sugar can be quite severe. This is why it is important to understand when to break a fast and when your fast might be hurting you rather than helping you.

- **Dizziness:** Many people are aware of the fact that fasting can lead to dizziness. Usually, this is a symptom that lessens over time as you become comfortable with fasting; however, dizziness is usually an indicator that you are either dehydrated or need to break your fast for your own health.
- **Weakness:** During a fast, one can feel weak as they walk, pick things up, or otherwise navigate life. This is normal for the first few fasts, but if you feel like you cannot function at all, something is wrong.
- **Loss of muscle mass:** Sometimes, those who fast can experience a loss of muscle mass, but this isn't usually the fault of fasting itself; rather, this happens due to not eating enough protein during your feeding windows. In Chapter 3, we discussed the importance of eating enough protein. Be sure to revisit that guidance if you need help with protein or consult your doctor.

Because fasting can have some effects like the ones mentioned, understanding how to personalize your schedule and fasting routine is vital. With this understanding, you can be sure that fasting is helping—and not hurting—you and your ability to reach your goals.

In order to avoid potentially life-threatening impacts from a fast—or even to simply avoid unhealthy and unpleasant experiences—be sure to talk to your doctor beforehand. You should ask them questions like what fasting options are best for you, what benefits you personally can gain, and how you can ensure nutritional balance while fasting. If you are choosing to go with

5:2 fasting, be sure to ask what they think a good calorie limit would be for you on those two fasting days.

Now that you understand the impacts of fasting on health and vice versa, it is time to get into the nitty-gritty of the best way to prevent such impacts from ruining your fasting journey. Let's talk about personalizing your fasting schedule now.

PERSONALIZING YOUR SCHEDULE

One of the best things that you can do in order to truly make your fast enjoyable is to personalize it. Not only does personalizing your fast make it a more pleasant experience, but it can help mitigate health risks from fasting as well. In this section, we are going to talk about the importance of personalizing your fasting schedule and the different options that you have for personalizing the fasting options mentioned at the beginning of the chapter.

Why Personalize Your Fasting Schedule?

For some reason, a lot of people seem to believe that when you personalize a fast or modify fasting techniques, it is "cheating." The thing about that mentality is that you cannot cheat on a fast unless you are eating during the fasting window, and even then, "cheating" can be warranted for your safety! Otherwise, modifying a fasting technique, window, strategy, or rule to fit your needs and lifestyle is perfectly fine. With that being said, why should you bother personalizing your fast?

For starters, personalizing your fast accounts for individual variability and needs. In other words, customizing your fast can help you achieve what you want out of fasting by making the structure of it your own. This is especially important because everyone responds to fasting and fasting techniques differently. Due to medical issues, lifestyle choices, and even genetics, fasting is not going to be an equal experience for everyone who participates. When you personalize the experience, it can be comfortable and effective, *and* help you to meet your goals.

Additionally, personalization takes into consideration medical needs and medication usage. There are a lot of medications that you have to take with food, medical conditions that require food during certain times of day, and other aspects of life that can make fasting quite challenging for some people. This is where customizing your fast can be a superhero in disguise.

Beyond that, customizing your fast empowers you to keep up with a lifestyle you enjoy. You do not have to change your exercise routine, brunch schedule, social activities, and other aspects of your life just to fit fasting in, so long as you are open to personalization. Personalizations like low calories during 5:2 fasting or adjusted fasting windows can be a lifesaver in such cases.

Ultimately, there is not really a strong reason that supports a lack of customization within fasting—in fact, it is quite the opposite. With that being said, let's delve into what you can do to truly make any fasting schedule your own.

Customizing a 5:2 Fast

Let's begin by taking a look at how you can customize 5:2 fasting, as this is the easiest to customize yet simultaneously has the most questions surrounding it. When you work with 5:2 fasting, you have a lot of options for personalization, including

- **Adjusting calorie intake:** Some people choose to completely fast for two 24-hour periods every week during 5:2 fasting. This can seem daunting or truly impossible for some individuals. You can choose to eat 500–600 calories on such days, which is the default, but you can even raise this amount in accordance with specific dietary needs.
- **Pick your fasting days wisely:** 5:2 fasting should be done with two separate days in mind, not two days back to back. With that being said, you have the power to select your two days as days that are the easiest for you, such as days when you are off work or have no commitments.
- **Emphasize hydration:** Rather than lament the fact that you are not eating, try to make the focus of your fasting days hydration. In other words, embrace the opportunity to hydrate through water, sugar-free juices, noncaffeinated teas, and more. This will help your fast be less mentally taxing.

Beyond that, do not hesitate to ask your doctor how a 5:2 fast can be more accommodating to your specific needs.

Customizing Time-Restricted Fasts

Both 16/8 and 14/10 fasting options classify as time-restricted fasts, because they limit the amount of time that you have within a day to fast. This can be troubling for individuals with specific dietary needs, medication habits, and so on, but the good news is that you can also customize a time-restricted fast. Some of the ways that you can do so include

- Personalize your feeding window based on your lifestyle. Something a lot of people believe is that sleeping during a fast does not count, but it totally does! The time you spend sleeping is time you spend not eating. Depending on your lifestyle, you can set it up so that your fasting window follows different arrangements, such as

  - If you sleep from 10 p.m. to 6 a.m., you can fast from 6 p.m. to 10 a.m. if you are more active in the middle of the day.
  - For morning people, you can start your fast at midday.
  - Night owls may opt for breaking their fast in the afternoon.

- Play around with duration. While 16/8 and 14/10 fasting windows are the most common, you can start with a 12-hour fasting window and gradually move those times around to find what is most comfortable for you. Just because the fasting hours you choose are not "established" or mentioned in this book does not mean that they cannot be effective and valid!
- Prioritize nutrients. To help you stay fuller longer and avoid health risks, be sure to prioritize nutrient-rich food during your feeding windows.

Beyond that, you can also personalize your fasting experience by

- **Listening to your body:** If your body says that it is time to stop fasting, then it is time to stop. You can tell this is the case if you are having negative effects from a fast or particular challenges that make it hard to continue, then you may need to modify your fast or consider a different approach. Listen to your energy, mood, and well-being to help you decide.
- **Experimenting and adjusting:** Do not be afraid to change things up until you find what works best for you. Your first fasting strategy does not have to be the one that you maintain throughout the course of your journey.
- **Being mindful of long-term sustainability:** As you try out different options, think about what can be the most beneficial in the long term. If a method is only something you can handle for a few weeks—or even a few days—then it is not going to lead to a long-term practice that benefits your goals.

Consider your needs and prioritize them when you think about fasting; do not be afraid to make fasting your own, because, at the end of the day, you are fasting for yourself—not anyone else.

BREAKING YOUR FAST

In the last section, I mentioned the idea of "breaking a fast" several times. Now, it is time for us to focus on what breaking a fast is and how you can do so properly. To begin, what is breaking a fast? The term "breaking a fast" refers to the act of ending a fast by eating before your designated fasting period was meant to end. Most of the time, you will not end a fast just because you are hungry—ending a fast early is typically the result of experiencing a medical issue or complications that make continuing a fast less than beneficial.

However, you cannot just end a fast willy-nilly. Some people choose to end a fast by pigging out on a buffet, for example, which can truly eliminate any benefits that you just obtained. Simultaneously, breaking a fast with the wrong foods can be unsafe if you are experiencing a medical issue. Ending a fast the smart way, however, can be really beneficial: it can heighten nutrient absorption, improve digestive health, and regulate your blood sugar (among other things).

Breaking a fast can include different actions depending on the length of a fast. For example, breaking a short fast means that you should

- **Start with hydration.** Before you eat anything, have a glass of water to rehydrate and help your body get into digestive mode.
- **Eat a small yet balanced meal.** A balanced meal with protein, healthy fats, and carbohydrates will benefit you the most when it comes to breaking a fast.

- **Avoid sugar and processed foods.** Such foods can lead to blood sugar spikes that pose a health risk.

On the other hand, breaking a long fast is more beneficial if you

- **Break with a light meal.** A light meal that is easy to digest can be wonderful for breaking a longer fast and allowing your digestive system to begin working its magic once again.
- **Include probiotics.** Probiotic foods like yogurt or fermented vegetables can really help your gut health after a fast.
- **Try bone broth.** Many people enjoy ending a fast with bone broth, as it is easy to digest, provides nutrients, and is good for gut health.

Outside of those tips, it is also a good idea to know what kind of foods to break your fast with. Ideally, your first meal after a fast should contain strong sources of protein, healthy fats, complex carbohydrates, fruits and vegetables, and hydrating foods. You should make sure that you avoid overeating as well, especially after a long fast, to prevent medical complications and negate any positive effects of the fast.

MISTAKES TO AVOID

The first time you participate in a fast can be the hardest because there are tons of mistakes that beginners make on their fasting journey. While nobody is perfect, perhaps having some of those mistakes in mind will help you avoid them before they even come to your attention. Some of the common mistakes that beginners are prone to making on their journey include

- **Neglecting proper nutrition:** A big mistake that many people make is ending a fast with poor nutrition and not eating healthy foods during feeding windows. If you are not noticing significant results from your IF journey, then chances are, your nutritional choices could use some help. Make sure that you pay attention to guidelines for proper, balanced meals, and consult with your doctor if you are worried about making the right food choices.
- **Not eating enough during feeding windows:** Sometimes, those who fast opt to eat only a little during their feeding windows. While small meals are great to break a fast with, you have to eat enough during your feeding windows. If you do not, you run the risk of over-eating later or breaking your fast early.
- **Over-exercising:** It's a common misconception that exercising a lot during a fast is beneficial. While light exercise or exercise typical to your lifestyle can be beneficial, exercising in excess can actually put you at risk of health detriments.
- **Choosing the wrong program:** If your IF routine is not benefiting you, you might be on the wrong program. Give a different fasting routine a chance, or consult with your doctor to see what you can do to have the results that you desire.
- **Bumpy transition:** It's common to underestimate the value of a smooth transition from fasting to eating;

however, this transition is instrumental for the fasting routine you pick to have results! When you break your fast, make sure that you do so in a way that is smooth and mindful based on the information provided above.

- **Over-eating:** A lot of people think that fasting means that you can eat whatever you want, whenever you want. While fasting does make it easier to have some dietary freedoms during your eating windows, binge eating and overeating can make fasting nonbeneficial.

- **Too strict of a diet:** Sometimes, a lack of results can be due simply to the fact that you are being too hard on yourself. Make sure that you are eating enough and eating healthy foods, and that you are not holding 24-hour fasts more than twice a week.

- **Forgetting to hydrate:** Forgetting to hydrate and, therefore, becoming dehydrated puts you at risk of health concerns.

- **Not getting enough sleep:** Sleep is actually very important for intermittent fasting. When you get enough sleep, your body is able to digest, regulate, and process. Plus, sleeping through some of your fast makes it ten times easier!

Remember, your first try probably will not be perfect; if you make a mistake or two, do not sweat it! Just try harder next time, and all shall be well.

SUMMARY BOX

Before selecting your fasting window, be sure to

- consider your health status, medical conditions, and any medications you take.

- determine any time-based priorities you have, like work or social events, that may impact your fast.

- choose a plan that does not drastically influence your current lifestyle and routines.

The best methods for beginner intermittent fasting windows are

- **16/8 fasting:** Fasting for 16 of the 24 hours in a day.

- **14/10 fasting:** Fasting for 14 hours of the day.

- **5:2:** Fasting for two days out of the week.

For women over 50, finding the right intermittent fasting schedule is invaluable. Before you begin a new IF regimen, however, it's a good idea to consult with your doctor—and a must if you have any medical conditions or take any medications. With all of that information in your IF toolkit, you're probably wondering how IF can help you manage your weight. Well, wonder no longer; that's where we're headed with the next chapter.

MAKE A DIFFERENCE WITH YOUR REVIEW

Unlock the Power of Generosity

"The best exercise for the heart is reaching down and lifting someone else up."

— TIMOTHY PINA

To all my wonderful readers who believe in the power of giving:

Did you know that people who give selflessly often find more joy and satisfaction in life? That's what I've learned, and I'm committed to spreading that joy as far as I can.

Now, I have a special request for you...

Would you be willing to extend a helping hand to someone you've never met?

This person is a lot like you - perhaps where you were a few years ago or maybe even last week. They are eager to learn, longing to make positive changes in their life, especially when it comes to their health and well-being after 50, but not sure where to start.

Our goal is to make the knowledge of intermittent fasting for women over 50 accessible to everyone. Every step I take is directed towards this mission. But to truly reach everyone, I need your help.

You see, most people do judge a book by its cover and by its reviews. So, here's my heartfelt plea on behalf of a fellow woman over 50 who you've never met:

Please consider leaving a review for this book.

This simple act, which costs nothing and takes just a moment, could be a life-changing gift for another woman. Your review could help another:

...woman over 50 feel more energetic and healthy.

...grandmother keep up with her grandkids.

...professional woman maintain her health in a hectic world.

...individual discover the joy of healthy living.

...dream of a healthier, happier life become a reality.

To share your thoughts and help someone in need, it's easy and quick: just leave a review.

Please scan the QR code below to leave your review:

If the idea of helping someone you've never met brings a smile to your face, then you're exactly the kind of person I wrote this book for. Welcome to our community of caring, strong women over 50.

I'm excited to continue to support you in your journey to better health and well-being with the strategies and insights in the upcoming chapters.

Thank you deeply. Now, let's get back to our journey together.

Your biggest fan, Kevin Sterling

PS - Remember, sharing knowledge is one of the greatest gifts. If you think this book can help another woman over 50, why not spread the love and recommend it to her? Your recommendation could be the start of her journey to a healthier, happier life.

5

THE SCALE AND BEYOND— MANAGING WEIGHT

M any sources indicate that intermittent fasting can be just as effective as calorie counting when it comes to weight loss. Depending on the type of fasting that you do, you can lose, on average, between three percent and eight percent of your starting weight thanks to fasting. For countless people, their main goal of IF is to lose weight. That's why this chapter centers itself around helping you with key strategies that can lead to effective weight management due to IF.

UNDERSTANDING MENOPAUSAL WEIGHT GAIN

As mentioned in Chapter 2, a common side effect of menopause is weight gain. This happens due to fluctuations in hormones, eating patterns, metabolic rate, and more, and it is a quite normal side effect of menopause. But something being common does not mean that it is desirable, and for many women over 50, weight gain is one of the worst symptoms imaginable.

Beyond simply despising age-related weight gain, there are countless health benefits associated with maintaining a healthy weight:

- **Reduced blood pressure:** One of the more favorable benefits associated with maintaining a healthy weight is reduced blood pressure. High blood pressure can contribute to numerous health issues, including increasing your risk of various diseases and health conditions as well. Beyond that, high blood pressure can reduce the activities you participate in and medications you can take and can otherwise restrict your life.
- **Improved muscle mass:** A healthy weight inherently means that you have less fat in your body, which means there is more room for muscle. Beyond that, the practices people engage with that lead to healthy weight —including exercise and fasting—can help improve muscle mass. Unhealthy weight—both under and overweight levels—is also associated with lower/reduced muscle mass.
- **Improved blood sugar levels:** Because those with healthier weights tend to balance their sugar intake more carefully and have better insulin sensitivity, they are more likely to have healthy blood sugar levels. Poor blood sugar levels can be associated with diabetes and other life-threatening health conditions.

- **Improved cholesterol levels:** Eating right and maintaining a healthy weight means that you are less likely to have unhealthy levels of cholesterol—which means that you are also less likely to suffer from heart attack, stroke, and other health concerns.
- **Improved mobility:** Overweight individuals often have problems with mobility, including being unable to carry out daily tasks like bathing, playing with children, or getting to work with ease. Even underweight people experience mobility issues. However, a healthy weight will allow you to move freely without pain or restriction.
- **Enhanced mental health:** It might not be apparent how weight ties into mental health, but those with a healthy weight are less likely to feel the effects of depression, anxiety, stress, self-esteem issues, and more.
- **Less joint pain:** Both overweight and underweight individuals suffer from an excess of joint pain, making it hard to function day in and day out. One of the most simple yet effective ways to minimize this pain is through maintaining a healthy weight.
- **Decreased risk of most cancers, diabetes, heart disease, and stroke:** By losing weight or maintaining a healthy weight, your body can heal or destroy damaged cells that result in the development of such medical issues.
- **Decreased risk or improvement in osteoarthritis and sleep apnea:** Excessive weight is often linked with sleep problems, osteoarthritis, and other risks that can lower your quality of life.

Beyond that, menopause can also contribute to unhealthy weight gain. In and of itself, unhealthy weight gain has myriad health risks that accompany it. There are countless severe health dangers that stem from neglecting unhealthy weight gain, including but not limited to

- pancreatitis
- stroke
- gout
- coronary artery disease
- hypertension
- cataracts
- gallbladder disease
- venous diseases
- urinary incontinence
- nonalcoholic fatty liver disease
- osteoarthritis
- diabetes
- mental health disorders
- obstructive sleep apnea
- most kinds of cancer
- hypoventilation syndrome

Knowing this, it becomes a desire *and* a necessity to maintain a healthy weight—but how can you do that? The secret to maintaining a healthy weight through weight management or loss is none other than our best friend, intermittent fasting.

FASTING AS A WEIGHT MANAGEMENT TOOL

Intermittent fasting is one of the safest, fastest, and most widely recommended ways for women above 50 to lose weight. Not only is intermittent fasting an excellent tool that almost anyone can use, but it utilizes several different strategies and changes to optimize how much weight you lose, thanks to an IF practice.

In particular, when done properly, intermittent fasting means that you are eating fewer calories in a day. The idea is not to make up for missed meals—it is to fast through those meals and then continue to eat as normal during feeding windows. Moreover, the psychological changes and habits picked up through intermittent fasting can leave you with a far healthier relationship with food.

In order to maximize your weight loss and other benefits as a result of intermittent fasting, one of the most important things to do is keep in mind several strategies. The first of those strategies is to identify your weight loss goals. Are you working to lose 5 pounds or 50? This makes a drastic difference in what fasting methods you can use and how fast you will see results. By understanding what your goal for IF is, you will find far more success through learning strategies and maintaining motivation.

Furthermore, it is important to stick to ideal calorie needs while remaining healthy. If you should be eating normally five days of the week and eating 500–600 calories on two days, stick to that plan. Do not shoot to eat zero calories on fast days, and definitely do not try to eat 500–600 calories every single day of the week. That is the line where fasting goes into starvation, which is both ineffective for weight gain and life-threatening. On the flip side, be sure that you are not going *over* your calorie needs either. A fasting habit will not work for weight loss if you interchange fasting with binge eating!

I also highly recommend that you sit down and figure out a meal plan. We went over how you can do so already, but there are so many benefits of meal planning for IF that we cannot *not* talk about it again! Meal planning takes loads of stress out of the process of intermittent fasting, and beyond that, it can also help you account for calorie needs, macro- and micronutrient balances, and more, all ahead of time. When you have a meal plan, you do not have to be confined to what you eat either. You have the power to choose your own meals and even to plan that outing with your friends into your meal plan. Sounds like freedom to me!

And because you are on an eating plan that inherently involves fewer calories than you are used to, it is also important that you make the calories that you do eat count. Rather than consuming a 500-calorie meal that consists of Doritos, Coke, and a frozen hamburger, try to balance your meals more appropriately. That's not to say that you can never have a treat or junk food, but you should have those foods in moderation—and never break a fast with them.

A lot of people are concerned about how they can still eat three meals a day without skipping meals, which is a valid concern; skipping meals entirely is not healthy! Instead of skipping meals altogether, I always recommend trying a smaller breakfast, a bigger lunch, and a smaller dinner. This does two things. First, it provides you with enough energy to navigate your day while still keeping you full throughout. Second, it helps you start and end your daily fasts with light meals that are fulfilling but easy to digest. You can fit your treats and junk food into that schedule accordingly, but it is a good idea to avoid breaking a fast with high sugar or processed foods. Plus, entering a fast on a stomach full of nutrient-packed foods is going to do you well.

The last tip that I have for you when it comes to getting the most out of intermittent fasting and weight loss is to never, ever break a fast with caffeine. While a tasty iced coffee or even a black coffee might seem like a good treat after a challenging fast, the caffeine itself can dehydrate you, resulting in weight retention. Beyond that, the sugar in caffeinated drinks can spike your insulin levels, which makes the effects of a fast wear off far quicker. This means that for the most successful weight loss, it is best to end your fast with water.

EMOTIONAL EATING

Many people experience emotional eating. While common, emotional eating can serve as a major roadblock between you and the weight management goals you are hoping for. In order to help you toss emotional eating habits in the trash once and for all, it is important to understand not just what emotional eating is, but why you do it and how to stop it in its tracks as well.

Simply put, emotional eating involves eating to handle particularly difficult emotions. For many people, emotional eating and binge eating—where one consumes far more calories than one needs in a short period of time—are synonymous. Those who habitually eat to cope with their emotions follow a typical cycle that can look something like

- **Emotional trigger:** Something upsets you or makes you feel a strong emotion that is overwhelming, unfamiliar, or painful.
- **Coping skills fail:** Any healthy coping skills you may know of do not kick in, resulting in you turning to food.
- **Emotional eating:** You eat in order to deal with those feelings, often eating past the point of fullness and consuming unhealthy or comforting foods.
- **Dopamine spike:** Temporarily, the rush of unhealthy or comforting foods and the comfort that eating brings can alleviate the pain you started out with.
- **Guilt, sadness, or shame:** Many people who emotionally eat feel guilt or similar negative emotions surrounding their unhealthy coping skill. This results in a blow to self-esteem.

And this gets repeated every time there is an emotional trigger.

It is an unfortunate cycle that can lead to an unhealthy relationship with food, weight gain, and even severely unhealthy conditions and medical issues. However, no one overeats or emotionally eats without reason, even if that reason is buried deep. Why do *you* emotionally eat?

There are five common reasons that people form a habit of turning to emotional eating:

1. **Stress:** Stress is one of the top reasons that people blame for overeating. When stressed out, it is likely that you are apt to confuse stress with hunger, or that the comfort of eating can seem to bring peace.
2. **Stuffing emotions:** The idea of emotional eating is conjoined with the idea that you can "stuff" your emotions down through food. For some people, stuffing their emotions works temporarily; however, those emotions inevitably pile up and lead to more and more emotional eating in the long run.
3. **Boredom or feelings of emptiness:** Sometimes, emotional eating is as simple as being bored. For others, emotional eating is a way to satiate feelings of emptiness, replacing that emotional emptiness with physically feeling full.
4. **Childhood habits:** For a lot of people, emotional eating begins in childhood. This can be due to the fact that parents did not encourage healthy eating habits, or due to the fact that emotional eating was used to replace parental figures due to neglect.
5. **Social influence:** Social eating, parties, and even influential advertising can introduce us to poor habits and unhealthy products that inevitably become a focal point of emotional eating.

To really dig into your personal motivations for emotional eating, some questions you might ask yourself include

- Do you feel powerless or out of control around food?
- Do you eat when you are not hungry or when you are full?
- Do you eat to feel better?
- Do you reward yourself with food?
- Do you eat more when you are feeling stressed?
- Does food make you feel safe? Do you feel like food is a friend?
- Do you regularly eat until you've stuffed yourself?

With that being said, there is a silver lining to all of this. You have the power to change your emotional eating habits right here and now. If you find yourself beginning or participating in emotional eating habits, I want you to simply notice those feelings and behaviors without judgment—judging yourself makes you more likely to engage with unhealthy coping mechanisms like emotional eating in the first place. Once you've done that, you can work with one or more of the following skills to replace emotional eating with a healthier method of coping:

- **Do not deprive yourself.** Sometimes, those who eat emotionally pick foods that they consider to be "bad" foods for their eating session. The easiest way to stop this habit is by refusing to deprive yourself of food. For instance, if you commonly binge on Oreos, try having one or two as a snack, treat, or with your meal. Associate that food with neutral emotions and make it something you are "allowed" to have, and slowly, it will not be a comfort object during emotional times.

- **Soothe your stress.** If stress is your reason for emotional eating, then mastering some strong coping mechanisms for stress can be the key to overcoming emotional eating. Easier said than done, I know, but self-improvement does take work.
- **Keep an emotional eating journal.** You can use an emotional eating journal to track the time, date, trigger, and contents of your emotional eating session. While such a practice might feel upsetting or shameful, it can eventually empower you to understand patterns that can be broken.
- **Find another way to feed your feelings.** If you feel like emotional eating, try something else. Consider painting your emotions, exercise them away, take a warm bath, or try anything else healthy that allows you to express your emotions and satisfy them.
- **Take away temptation.** If you truly cannot avoid eating certain foods due to cravings and habits, just refuse to buy those foods. Do not keep the rest of what you have until it is gone; throw it away or donate it. Taking away temptation means that you have to find another outlet, even if it is healthy food.
- **Learn from setbacks.** The age-old adage that everyone makes mistakes could not be truer. However, you do not have to let those mistakes define your life moving forward. Instead, learn from those mistakes, discover what you did wrong that resulted in emotional eating, and strive to do better next time.

- **Snack healthy.** Snacking on healthy foods is good for you, can keep you full, and is a wonderful way to discourage emotional eating.

Mindful Eating

Now that we've talked about emotional eating in detail, it is important to consider its powerful opposite—mindful eating. While emotional eating can contribute to weight gain and health problems, mindful eating has been linked to weight management as well as increased satisfaction with food and meals. It is one of the best ways to form a powerful, healthy relationship with food—but what *is* mindful eating in the first place?

Think back to your last meal for just a second. What did you have? What were you doing while you ate? Can you remember how the food existed on your plate with all five senses? Chances are, you do not remember the intricate details of your meal. And while every meal cannot be memorable, the idea of mindful eating is less about memory and more about the experience—if you cannot remember the details of your last meal, you probably did not have much of an experience.

With that said, mindful eating involves being in the present moment as you eat your food. It is something so small and so overlooked, yet so powerful at the same time. When you spend time with your food through mindful eating, you gain respect for your food, fill up faster due to paying attention to hunger cues, and so much more. You can hone the skill of mindful eating by

- **Honor your food.** Think about all of the good things that your food does for you. It nourishes your body, gives you energy, helps you bond with others, and so much more. Eating is a wonderful time to show appreciation for your food, which improves mood, mindfulness, and appreciation. Honor your food by thinking about gratitude toward your food, appreciating the experience you have with it, and other similar thoughts.
- **Engage the senses.** As you eat, try to make it a habit of engaging all five of your senses with your food. This way, you have a memorable experience with each meal and are surely present. Discover what you can observe via sight, taste, texture, smell, and maybe even hearing if the meal makes a sound somehow.
- **Serve modest portions.** You can always go back for more if you are still hungry, so why not serve modest portions? When there is less on your plate, you can give targeted attention and focus to each and every bite, truly appreciating your meals for what they are.
- **Chew well and in small bites.** Mindful eating does not stop just because the food is in your mouth. Take small bites and chew those bites well, savoring the flavor and texture of the food as you do. This helps further your appreciation for the food, *and* your thorough chewing improves digestion.

With these tips, you can really begin a habit of mindful eating that benefits you. In the context of intermittent fasting, mindful eating can help you make the most out of each meal, improve digestion, and avoid overeating as you close out your fast. All around, it is a wonderful technique that can empower you to have a healthier, more appreciative relationship with your food and body.

Beyond the Scale

For a lot of people, the most important measure of weight loss success is the scale. So many people live and die by the number on the scale. What if I told you that the scale is far from the most important factor to consider on your weight loss journey? It is true! Just because the number on the scale is not changing does not mean that you have not experienced changes in your body or made progress. The reality of the situation is that there are numerous ways to determine progress, none of which involve the scale.

For example, a trusty tape measure can be your best friend. The number on the scale does not really mean anything in a practical sense. The number on the scale does not show how well you fit your clothes, how healthy you are, or even how much progress you've made in many cases. However, a tape measure can be helpful when you consider the distribution of your weight, especially if you have goals specific to parts of the body, i.e., toning your arms. With a tape measure, you may see slower progress from week to week, but it is another reliable method that can replace the scale.

In addition, you can use how well a certain article of clothing fits to measure your progress. In fact, I think fitting into a certain item of clothing is a far more realistic, motivational, and positive goal than achieving a numerical weight. For instance, if you have a goal to get to 140 pounds, you might get to that weight and realize you are not happy with your progress—maybe you've lost too much, too little, or do not look how you expected you would. Instead, fitting into a pair of jeans that are one or two sizes smaller can have tangible effects and success that you see and feel.

You can also measure your success with weight loss based on the quality of aspects of your life. Remember that your weight loss goals do not have to be all about the numbers. For example, weight loss can often bring about improved energy levels. This might be your goal! If you notice that your energy levels are improving, then you are doing well. You can also measure your success based on mobility, quality of sleep, how well you stuck to a meal plan, and other similar things.

Strength is another valuable way to measure weight loss and health goals. As I mentioned earlier, those with high or unhealthy weights tend to struggle significantly with strength as a result of lowered muscle mass or health. As you lose weight, especially through exercise and eating right with IF, you can track progress by determining how much stronger you've gotten using objective measures like weights.

30-Day Photo Progress Challenge

As you embark upon IF for weight loss or weight management, something you can do to track your progress besides hawk-eyeing the scale is to take photos. Every day for 30 days, try taking a photo of yourself that shows most of your body in good lighting. This way, while you may not notice results from Monday to Tuesday, you'll have a record *and* will be able to notice the extended results from a month of work.

Journaling Prompts

Alongside the photo challenge, I recommend working with journaling prompts to reflect, track progress, and manage how you feel. Some journal prompts you can use include

- Before you begin, consider what you hope to capture in your 30-Day Photo Progress Challenge. What specific progress do you want to document? Is it related to a personal goal, a skill you're developing, a physical transformation, or perhaps the growth of a project from start to finish?
- After the first week of photos, reflect on what you've noticed that you hadn't seen before. How has the act of taking daily photos changed your perspective on the progress you are making?
- Halfway through the challenge, think about the obstacles you've encountered. Have there been days when you didn't see any progress or days when taking a photo felt like a chore? How did you overcome these challenges?
- As you approach the latter part of the challenge, focus on the present moment within your journey. How has this daily practice of documenting progress kept you grounded or mindful? Have you found yourself more engaged in the process or activity you are capturing?

- On the last day, take time to reflect on the overall experience. What have you learned about yourself and your ability to commit to a 30-day challenge? How do the images collectively represent your journey, and what story do they tell about the progress you've made?

Summary Box

Emotional eating is a major contributor to weight gain for women. Emotional eating can be avoided by

- Refuse to deprive yourself of the food you enjoy.

- Soothe your stress in other ways.

- Keep a journal that pertains to your emotional eating habits.

- Feed your feelings without using food.

Intermittent fasting can be a wonderful way to achieve the benefits associated with weight loss and weight management. It makes up just one element of a holistic approach to weight loss, meaning that you shouldn't rely solely on IF to help you achieve the body of your dreams. However, I do encourage you to work with IF, tracking beyond the scale, and managing emotional eating for the best outcomes.

6

MOVEMENT MATTERS—SYNCING EXERCISE WITH INTERMITTENT FASTING

I t is well-recognized that both physical training and fasting have beneficial effects when it comes to health and overall body composition. For instance, aerobic training and fasting can work together as a team to strengthen muscle tissue while also reducing body fat mass. This means that exercise, when combined with intermittent fasting, serves as an indelible way to improve your health, manage weight, and achieve satisfaction. In this chapter, you'll find out how you can complement intermittent fasting with exercise, as well as what routines are the most effective for women over 50.

THE IMPORTANCE OF EXERCISE

When it comes to exercise, you may be filled with dread. Getting hot and sweaty is not fun, and what is exercise good for anyway? But as it turns out, exercise is more important than ever for women over the age of 50. Just a few of the benefits of exercise for women over the age of 50 include

- **Bone health:** Bone health is an important health aspect for women over 50, particularly because menopause can reduce bone health. Exercise can be a powerful tool for improving the health and strength of your bones. As a result, this can reduce your risk of injury or the development of bone-related medical issues.

- **Muscle health:** Exercise naturally works with the muscles, another part of the body that can decline in health with age. When you exercise—specifically strength training—it can improve the health and resilience of your muscles. Like bone health, muscle health can reduce the risk of injury and improve your satisfaction with life overall.

- **Energy levels:** Exercise improves energy levels. It's a known fact. And everyone, especially those over 50, can do with a natural boost of energy. Thanks to exercise, you can successfully combat low energy levels that accompany both age and fasting. This means that you do not have to rely on caffeine or other unhealthy options that can lower the quality of your fasts.

- **Metabolism:** Metabolism slows down as you age, but exercise is the secret to kick-starting it back up. This can help with weight loss, weight management, energy, nutrient absorption, and much more, improving one of the most pressing symptoms of aging that many women deal with.

- **Strength:** For a lot of women over 50, strength is a challenge. You might feel weak or shaky performing daily activities, or you may feel as though you cannot handle tasks that used to be easy for you. The solution to all of this is simple: exercise. Exercise is a phenomenal way to build up strength.
- **Balance:** Balance might not feel like a big issue, but it is something we use every single day. With exercise, you can balance far better and maintain balance for longer, improving your quality of life.
- **Weight loss:** Last and most definitely not least, exercise is wonderful for weight loss. It burns extra calories, makes your body work harder, and helps you achieve various health benefits while losing weight.

Moreover, exercise during IF can be beneficial when it comes to autophagy. Autophagy is when the cells of your body and bodily processes are able to clear out damaged or dead cells. This can impact aesthetic aspects of your life, like appearance, but most notably, autophagy is important because it can prevent the development of cancer and other diseases. Damaged or defunct cells create cancer, which means that boosting autophagy through IF and exercise can truly save your life.

In a sense, exercise and intermittent fasting are a dynamic duo that creates anti-aging effects. Every single one of the benefits I mentioned above counteracts what aging does to the body and mind, which means that through exercise and IF, you can find revitalized and youthful health, even after the age of 50.

WARMING UP, COOLING DOWN

When taking a look at exercise, you might think that speeding through or skipping a warm-up or cool-down is better; it gets you to the meat and potatoes of the exercise routine, after all. However, warming up and cooling down are not just important for the flow of the exercises; they are important to your health, safety, and ability to attain benefits from exercise. So, what is a warm-up, and what is a cool-down?

A warm-up happens before you exercise. Prior to diving into an exercise routine, you need to warm up. A warm-up exercise gradually increases your heart rate, blood circulation, and body temperature, preparing your body for more intense movement. This can reduce your risk of injury, as well as make your exercises more effective. On the other hand, cooling down refers to a process of allowing your body to slowly return to a resting state after exercise. This helps prevent soreness and aid in recovery.

There are many distinct benefits of engaging with warm-ups and cool-downs as a woman over 50:

- **Injury prevention:** Warming up allows more blood to flow to the muscles before you even begin to exercise. The result of that blood flow is better flexibility and strength, allowing you to avoid injury through proper preparation. Cooling down prevents injuries from developing after exercise by reducing stiffness and muscle soreness—all thanks to the gradual rest cooling down allows for.

- **Improved performance:** Warming up prepares your body for what it is going to face during exercise. It lets the body know to get ready, and as a result, you will experience optimized muscle function, coordination, reaction times, and more. This can make your workout more effective. Cooling down can help your after-workout performance improve as well by avoiding the abrupt cessation of intense physical activity.
- **Enhanced flexibility:** Both warming up and cooling down enhance your flexibility and range of motion, allowing for easier living and better health.
- **Heart rate regulation:** Warming up gradually increases your heart rate, and cooling down gradually decreases it. This means that your heart is never going from a resting state to your highest heart rate, or vice versa. Doing so is quite dangerous, underlining further the value of warming up and cooling down.
- **Mental preparation:** Finally, warm-up and cool-down exercises can allow you time to mentally prepare for exercise, working out with more motivation and appreciation.

Warm-Up Exercises

Now that you understand the importance of warming up and cooling down, you probably want to know *how* you can do so. Here are three of the best warm-ups for women over 50:

1. **March in place:** For this exercise, all you have to do is pretend you are a soldier marching! Get those knees up high and swing those arms to improve your heart rate, circulation, and muscle preparation.

2. **Arm circles:** With your arms parallel to the floor and aligned with your shoulders, simply make small arm circles. As you go, increase the size of those circles, then do the same thing in the opposite direction.

3. **Leg swings:** Hold onto a sturdy surface and allow your leg to swing from the hip, as though it is the hinge of a door. Swing both legs for a few moments, going front to back and then side to side to warm up your hips and legs.

Cool-Down Exercises

You cannot forget about cooling down! Here are three cool-down ideas you can use as well:

1. **Neck and shoulder stretch:** Gently tilt your head to one side, bringing your ear toward your shoulder. Hold this position for 15–30 seconds and then repeat on the other side. Follow this up with some shoulder rolls to release tension.

2. **Seated forward bend:** Sit on the floor with your legs straight out in front of you. Reach forward toward your toes, keeping your back straight, and hold the position for 15–30 seconds.

3. **Calf stretch:** Stand facing a wall and place one foot forward and the other back with the heel on the

ground. Lean forward, keeping the back leg straight, to stretch the calf muscles.

STRENGTH TRAINING 101

Strength training is one particular type of exercise that women over 50 can benefit from. It involves working out the muscles and other strength structures within the body to improve, you guessed it, strength. This is particularly beneficial to you because it can counteract some of the negative impacts of age—like weakness, muscle loss, and bone loss.

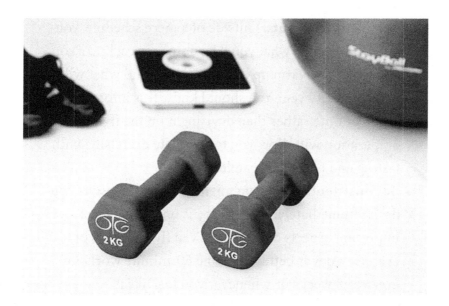

You might be wondering whether you can strength train while doing intermittent fasting. You definitely can! With the proper safety precautions and levels of understanding, IF and exercise at the same time can be safe and beneficial. To combine IF and strength training, you should

- **Set a schedule.** Setting a schedule is a must for anyone who wants to strength train alongside fasting. So, not only do you need a fasting schedule, but you need a strength training schedule as well. You'll find out more about what you should include as you go through this section!

- **Eat nutrient-dense food.** Eating food full of nutrients is important to fasting and strength training at the same time. When you exercise, your body needs more nutrients. Beyond that, the nutrients are helpful for IF benefits and exercise benefits, like increasing muscle mass.

- **Plan your workouts.** Outside of a mere schedule, you also have to plan what you'll be doing for each workout. How will you warm up and cool down, and what will you do in between? You should know this information ahead of time rather than devising it on the fly; preparation will allow you to correlate exercising with fasting and nutrition seamlessly.

- **Be consistent.** While you might not see the results you desire immediately, consistency is one of the most important aspects of exercise. Even five minutes of exercise a day is better than one 50-minute workout every 6–8 weeks or whenever you feel like it.

Strength training is not something that you can go into without some precautions in mind. A lot of beginners make mistakes, which means that you have the chance to learn from those mistakes before you make them. Some mistakes to watch out for include

- **Not eating enough:** Not eating enough is a common mistake people make when they first start training. Exercising intensely and regularly means that you need more nutrients, especially protein. Skipping out on nutrients can mean that your workouts actually cause muscle *loss*, not gain.

- **Overtraining:** Training too much can be dangerous. The body needs rest to solidify the work you are doing, and overexercising can put you at risk while fasting as well. It's a good idea to stick to three or four workout sessions a week max, with active recovery days (walking, light yoga) between, and one or two total rest days worked in.

- **Not adjusting workout intensity:** Strength training involves different intensities. If you truly cannot lift something, the intensity should be adjusted; struggling is dangerous and demotivating. Beyond that, if something has become too easy for you, you need to adjust the intensity so that you get the most out of your workout.

- **Not tracking progress:** As you exercise, it is important to monitor your progress in objective ways. Measuring muscle mass or using other measures mentioned for weight management in Chapter 5 can be helpful in showing you if you are doing well or if you need to change your methods for results.

- **Not consulting a professional:** Lastly, I recommend that you consult with a professional to ensure that you will not hurt yourself and that it is safe for you to engage in strength training. This goes especially for those with heart conditions, diabetes, or similar medical issues or medication needs.

Strength Training Exercises

Now, let's get you started with some of the best strength training exercises for your particular age, goals, and desires:

- **Push-ups:** Push-ups are particularly awesome because all you need is yourself. Your body weight serves as the weight you are working with, which means you do not need any fancy equipment. This works the upper body, and the exercise itself is modifiable for all needs!
- **Squats:** Similar to push-ups, squats leverage your body weight as a weight to work with. Working your lower body, core, and balancing skills, squats are also accessible, fun, and free to do.
- **Lunges:** Lunges are a versatile way to work the lower body and have fun at the same time. This exercise can be potentially beneficial for mobility in daily life, like when you are climbing the stairs, for instance.
- **Bicep curls:** Light weights can be used for bicep curls, strengthening your upper body muscles and improving mobility. You do not even need to buy weights—full water bottles, books, or other household items can be wonderful weights!

For some people, strength training exercises might still be too intense to start with. You do have some other options to help you get ready for strength training and get your body used to exercise. Cycling, yoga, and gentle Pilates can help you adjust to what it is like to exercise, strengthen your body, and more. Make sure to monitor your progress with these workouts as well.

GETTING STARTED WITH CARDIO

In addition to strength training, cardio can do wonders for improving your health and experience with intermittent fasting through exercise. Cardio exercises are any exercises that elevate the rate of your heart into your target heart rate range through rhythmic activity. Usually, this involves the use of oxygen to do so.

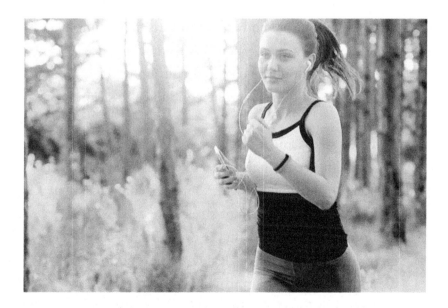

There are many benefits to cardio workouts for women over 50:

- **Strengthens muscles:** Cardio is another form of exercise that can counteract muscle weakness or loss due to age. Cardio can help you feel stronger and more stable, also boosting your confidence and well-being in the process.
- **Increases bone density:** Cardio also helps improve your bone density. Through exercises and the aerobic requirements of cardio, your bone density can strengthen and improve. This reduces age-related bone health issues, pain, and susceptibility to injury.
- **Improved sleep:** Exercise, in particular, is linked to improved sleep, but cardio specifically can take your sleep quality to the next level. When you get enough cardio exercise in, it is your body's clock. Cardio raises your internal body temperature, signifying that it is time to be awake. Then, you will have more energy throughout the day, and your body temperature will drop and be conducive to sleeping at night.
- **Reduced stress and anxiety:** Cardio is particularly beneficial for reducing stress and anxiety because it gets your endorphins pumping. Endorphins make it so that the body can handle pain or stress, and exercise is definitely putting stress on the body. But these boosted endorphins also help you deal with the emotional pain of anxiety and stress, improving your overall mood.
- **Strengthens heart and lungs:** Cardio gets your heart pumping and puts your lungs to work. This enhances the performance of your heart and lungs, letting you benefit from heart and lung health even while at rest.

Cardio is linked to the reduction of heart and lung-related medical ailments as well.

- **Increases metabolism:** Cardio exercise also enhances your metabolism. This means that your body processes food faster, aiding in weight and fat loss. Just remember to eat enough when you do cardio workouts.

And that's just the start of it.

There are numerous different cardio exercises that you can enjoy. One that I highly recommend is running. Running is free and accessible to most, and you can listen to music as well so there is no shortage of entertainment. As you run, be sure to consider appropriate warm-up and cool-down activities, hydration, nutrition, and more. A typical run for cardio should last about 15–20 minutes for beginners, but you can run longer or shorter depending on preference and fitness level. And if running is too strenuous for you right now, just start with a brisk walk! There's no shame in working to steadily build your aerobic capacity up over time.

Swimming is another good cardio workout that you can play around with. If you know how to swim, it is a fun workout that allows you to embrace the water. There are several swimming techniques to work different parts of the body, and you can even start out just treading water until you're comfortable. I recommend ensuring that you follow proper safety precautions, like not eating less than 30 minutes before swimming.

You also have other options like spin class, cycling, or climbing stairs. At the end of the day, cardio is cardio; there is nothing that says climbing up and down the stairs in your house cannot be as good as running a mile. Be sure to keep yourself hydrated and nourished as you engage with cardio workouts.

Balancing cardio with intermittent fasting is not very challenging, which is fortunate. I highly recommend that you save cardio for lighter workout days, focusing the harder ones on strength training. Still, cardio is not a proper rest day, so make sure that you rest in between workout days. Moreover, you should be sure to refuel with a good, balanced meal after your cardio workout.

BEST PRACTICES FOR EXERCISING WHILE FASTING

You can exercise while you are actively fasting, but you have to know how to do so safely. Exercising when you have not eaten in 16 hours, for instance, is not safe, nor is engaging with a particularly intense or rigorous routine on fasting days in 5:2 fasting. To keep yourself safe and allow the exercises to have the effect they are supposed to have—boosting your health—you have to keep in mind a few of the best practices for exercising while fasting.

First and foremost, it is important to think through the timing of both your exercise and fast. By now, you should know better than to schedule a rigorous exercise routine on a day when you are not eating very much. You also know better than to avoid exercising altogether. When it comes to truly empowering yourself through exercise and IF, it is important that you think through the timing. One of the best questions that you can ask yourself when it comes to considering timing is, "Is [day] good for [activity]?" It seems so simple, but so many people overlook that life-changing question.

Additionally, it is a good idea to select the exercises you prioritize based on macronutrient consumption. For example, muscle-related exercises are not going to work best if you are not eating a lot of protein on a particular day. If you do that, you run the risk of under-fueling your body for intense exercise, which puts you at risk of exhaustion and injury, among other things. Therefore, you have to consider what your body needs in terms of the macronutrients you should be consuming.

It's also wise to consider meal consumption and timing when exercise and IF are combined. For example, after a particularly rigorous exercise that uses a lot of muscle, it is a good idea to consume a balanced yet protein-rich meal to assist in building muscle. It's also smart to eat a balanced and nutritious meal 30–45 minutes prior to moderate or high-intensity exercise, as this can give you the energy and nutrients that you need for success. This means that you can start a fast just before exercising, exercise during your feeding window, or otherwise plan exercise and meals around one another.

Hydration is just as important as nutrition, especially when it comes to fasting while exercising. Because both fasting and exercise require intense calorie needs, you should make doubly sure that you are drinking enough water not just for being at rest, but for an intensely active day. Similarly, pay attention to your electrolytes, especially after you finish exercising. Exercise uses a ton of electrolytes, as you sweat profusely during even moderately intense workouts. A sports drink or other electrolyte-balancing option is perfect here.

When it comes to exercising in the middle of an active fast, you are not completely out of luck. Even if you have not eaten in a while, you can still safely consider exercise. The important factor here is to keep the intensity and duration of your exercise low. Light yoga or a peaceful walk is not going to hurt you, even on hour 10 of a 16-hour fast, for instance. Make sure that as you do exercise, you listen to your body, stop when you need to stop, and break your fast if you really need to.

At the end of the day, IF and exercise can be deeply entangled for a beautiful symphony of health. With the best practices mentioned above, as well as a consultation with a medical professional depending on your particular needs, you are golden when it comes to balancing IF and exercise for outstanding health results.

REST AND RECOVERY

It can seem as though in order to have the best health results, you have to work, work, work. And that's true, but probably not in the way you may think. Every moment, you are contributing to improving your health in some way. Fasting is contributing, exercise is contributing, but so is eating healthy, treating yourself once in a while, and resting and relaxing. Even when you are doing nothing, you are working toward your health. You do not have to hit the gym for six hours a day to be working on your health!

With that being said, it is important to highlight the value of rest and recovery when it comes to the exercise process. If you are doing strength training and cardio, there is no reason to exercise seven days a week. You absolutely need to take rest days as a part of self-care and improving your health, because rest days

- **Allow time for recovery.** Your body cannot recover from the strenuous exercise you are engaging in if you never give it the chance. If you continuously overwork your body without a break, all of the negative health consequences of age will worsen. In contrast, giving yourself time to recover enables your body to make those benefits really stick.
- **Prevent muscle fatigue.** If you stretch a rubber band long and hard enough, it'll eventually lose all of its elasticity. Your muscles are similar; working them constantly without giving them a break will cause your muscles to become fatigued. And when this happens, your muscles cannot work at optimal capacity, resulting in pain and weakness at *best.*
- **Reduce risk of injury.** When you rest your body in between workout days, your body has time to recuperate. This means that you can enter your workouts with a refreshed body ready to tackle a workout and *not* one that will collapse—literally— under pressure.
- **Improves performance.** Some people think that exercising everyday is how you can prevent your body from losing skill. In other words, people think that in

order to do 10 push-ups consistently, they have to do it every day. That's simply not true. Rest *improves* performance, not hinders it. From rest, you'll notice that you can not only still do 10 push-ups after rest, but you can do more and more as you exercise and rest interchangeably.

- **Supports healthy sleep.** Rest is also good for healthy sleep; you will not be kept up because of pain or inflammation, for instance. Rest also contributes to regulating your body's temperature and circadian rhythms.

Even if you feel like you can power through and exercise, your body might truly need a rest day. Fortunately, there are some objective signs you can look at and tell if your body needs a day or two off from exercise. For example, soreness, pain, and swelling mean that your body definitely needs a break. If you are feeling tired or fatigued, notice yourself doing less and less instead of more as you work out, or suffer from sleep problems, this can also indicate that you need a rest day.

Now, there are two ways to manage a rest day. One way is complete and total rest, which is great one to two times a week. But for active recovery days, the other type of rest, you can still move around, get some blood flowing, and let your body heal all while avoiding the feeling of being glued to the couch. On active rest and recovery days, movements like walking, gentle stretching, or light impact exercise can be a game-changer.

Summary Box

The best way to exercise in order to manage weight alongside fasting includes

- Warming up and cooling down
- Cardio
- Strength training
- Active recovery and rest days 1–3 times/week

Listening to your body is the most important thing when it comes to fitness through exercise. Just like it's important to find the right IF strategy for you, it's also important to find the right workout routine. Fitness is a journey, one that takes time, so don't be afraid to find what works for you and give it the time it needs to work. As we transition to the next chapter, you are going to uncover how to achieve mental clarity and emotional balance, thanks to IF.

PART IV

TOTAL WELLNESS

7

ACHIEVING MENTAL CLARITY
AND EMOTIONAL BALANCE

The mind is a powerful instrument. Every thought, every emotion that you create changes the very chemistry of your body.

— SADHGURU

The mind and body are intimately connected, whether that connection is immediately apparent to you or not. What you think about your body and the emotions you have take hold in physical ways, and the physical treatments that you subject your body to influence your mind as well. In this chapter, you'll come to understand the importance of taking care of your emotional and mental health, and how you can do so in the context of intermittent fasting.

STRESS MANAGEMENT

Stress is one of the most universal aspects of human life, as unfortunate as it is to say it. At one time or another, we have all experienced the tell-tale pangs of stress that indicate that something is going differently than we like—causing overwhelm, anxiety, or other hard-to-manage feelings. Stress can affect your body, and you cannot truly say that you've achieved a state of wellness until you can manage your stress healthily in the first place. This section is dedicated to helping you defeat stress as you venture toward self-improvement.

Many people can succinctly identify when they are stressed, but not many people are aware of the specific signs of stress. Half of the time, people do not even recognize that what they are experiencing is stress in the first place. Some of the common mental impacts of stress can include

- **Worry:** While a little worry will not hurt, it is not normal to be worried every moment of the day, or even for most of the day. Worrying to the point that it becomes impactful as a component of your life or that it takes up the majority of your day is a clear indicator of stress.
- **Anger:** Anger that is inexplicable or the result of having too much on your plate is another indication of stress. You might find yourself snapping or lashing out at others due to stress—a solid sign that you need better stress management techniques.

- **Depression:** Some people believe themselves to be depressed, when the actual culprit is not depression; it is stress cloaking itself as depression. Sometimes, the symptoms of stress look a lot like depression—lack of motivation, exhaustion, feeling down, and more.
- **Lack of focus:** Even when you have myriad tasks to focus on, stress can make focus a challenge. Your brain is working overtime, after all, so there is not much energy to expend focusing!

In addition, you may experience physical symptoms, such as

- **Headaches:** Stress can cause headaches. Emotional distress caused by stress is enough to do so on its own, but jaw clenching, dehydration, and lack of rest are other facets of stress that can lead to headaches as well.
- **Sleeping too much or too little:** Those who face chronic stress often suffer from insomnia, which can entail trouble falling or staying asleep. Some people, on the other hand, cope with stress by sleeping too much—even to the point it has severe consequences on their lives.
- **Upset stomach:** The body knows when the mind is in distress, and sometimes this can manifest as an upset stomach. When on a fasting journey, an upset stomach can be a dangerous thing!
- **Weight changes:** Stress can result in over or under-eating and metabolic changes, which can cause your weight to fluctuate in unhealthy ways.

- **Tension:** Lastly, stress makes you more prone to holding tension in your body. This can result in muscle tension and pain, jaw clenching, and more.

You might be thinking that you have no reason to be stressed or that you do not know why you are so stressed, but there are numerous causes of both long and short-term stress. And beyond that, you may not even know all of the different reasons behind your stress. Understanding the different causes of stress can benefit you in reducing stress. Some of those causes include

- having too much to do in too little of a timespan.
- having many small problems very close to each other, like being caught in traffic, spilling your coffee, and forgetting to send an email all in one day.
- preparing for a big event at work or school.
- having an argument or problems with work, home, or school.
- dealing with financial difficulties.
- suffering from long-term illness or caring for someone with one.

While it may be difficult to master, stress management is vital for anyone who hopes to have strong health and mental well-being. And as someone who participates in IF, your mental health is just as important as your physical health. Some of the best ways that you can manage stress—methods that I hope you will cultivate within your own life—are

- **Identify the source of your stress.** It might be challenging, but identifying why you feel so stressed can be vital to overcoming that stress in the first place. You can work to identify the source of your stress by considering what was going on before the stress became bad, and then slowly walking backward through events.

- **Start a stress journal.** Something you can do to get stressful emotions out of your head is to write those emotions down in a dedicated stress journal. Because your journal is private, this is the perfect place to rant about whatever you are experiencing. Plus, having a written record can enable you to notice trends and patterns in your stress.

- **Eliminate unhealthy coping mechanisms.** Managing stress inherently involves coping mechanisms, but you have to be able to break free from unhealthy coping mechanisms in order to heal. This means cutting out habits like overeating, bottling up emotions, and more so that those habits can be replaced with healthy coping tools.

- **Exercise.** Exercise is a positive and efficient way to manage stress. The resources offered in Chapter 6 can be a great help with using exercise for stress management in addition to the weight loss and IF benefits mentioned before!

- **Connect with others.** Stress relief can also come in the form of connecting with others, whether that's ranting to someone about your stress or simply spending quality, relaxing time with another human being. Human connection is inherently relaxing for many people.

- **Make time for fun.** Making time for fun and relaxing activities, even amidst a busy schedule, does wonders for reducing stress.
- **Master time management.** Chances are, your time management could use some work. Mastering basic time management techniques and strategies will be your best friend when it comes to defeating stress.

With all of that being said, stress management is not the only important consideration when it comes to managing your mental and emotional well-being. You also have to master emotional regulation!

EMOTIONAL REGULATION

Emotional regulation is a skill that anyone can hone, but few people take the time to develop. It involves being able to understand the emotions that you are feeling and handle them in a healthy way. With emotional regulation, you can understand and cope with your emotions in a way that is conducive to growth. You also do not have to worry about the negative impact of suppressed emotions thanks to emotional regulation superpowers.

It's interesting to note that fasting can impact your mood and emotions as well—and not always in a way that is positive.

Especially when you're new to the world of intermittent fasting, mood disturbances can be common. For instance, intermittent fasting lowers your blood sugar and can result in something called hypoglycemia. This can result in irritability, anxiety, and low levels of focus that make it hard to function in some respects during your first few fasts. Knowing this and the importance of emotional regulation overall, you're probably wondering what you can do to maintain emotional regulation both in and outside of your intermittent fasting journey.

First, it is important to learn how you can identify and reduce emotional triggers. An emotional trigger is a circumstance that results in heightened negative emotions, particularly sadness, distress, anxiety, or a similar feeling. After a trigger is presented, negative emotions—and often negative coping mechanisms—ensue. The way to prevent this loop is by identifying your triggers, which can feel overwhelming if you do not know how. I recommend keeping a log to analyze your triggers. Write down the time and date, what emotion you felt, and what happened just before it happened. Chances are, you've identified your trigger then and there. Similar triggers often bring about similar emotions, so take advantage of this knowledge to analyze patterns as well.

You should also be sure that you are focusing on the physical symptoms of emotions. Next time you are feeling a strong emotion, try tuning into how your body feels. You probably do not notice that anger speeds up your heart or that sadness feels like a discernible pang in your chest, but these physical indicators can be a great way to understand what you are feeling and how it impacts you. Moreover, tapping into physical indicators of an emotion is a very grounding experience. With such physical indicators, you can develop a profound understanding of your emotions and soothe physical ailments in a way that soothes emotional turmoil as well.

Another tactic for emotional regulation is to consider the story that you are telling yourself. For instance, it can be easy to get anxious about your partner coming home late from work. You might start thinking the worst—they are cheating, got into an accident, left you, and so on and so forth. This type of rumination is the "story" you are telling yourself, and almost always, that story is going to exacerbate whatever you are feeling. This applies to sadness, anger, stress, and all manner of emotions. Watch out for instances where you may be telling yourself that someone does not care for you or that you are a victim in particular; these are two stories that always lead to more assumptions and harm than needed.

In fact, rather than ruminating on your negative thoughts and emotions, I recommend working with positive self-talk. Self-talk refers to the way that we speak to ourselves and the stories we tell ourselves, and you have the ability to choose positive stories. The best method for learning how to engage with positive self-talk is to treat yourself like you would treat a friend in the same situation. Most people can admit that they would *never* speak to their friends how they speak to themselves in their own heads at times. Try to make the transition to treating yourself as you would a friend, and you'll notice that your mood and emotional regulation capabilities improve.

You should also know that you have a choice in how you respond. When emotions are high, particularly ones like anger or stress that result in lashing out, we feel as though we "have" to act in certain ways or that there is no other option. You *had* to lash out at your coworker for interrupting your task, right? Wrong! When you notice mental distress coming on, simply remind yourself that you do have a choice in how you respond, and you are 100% responsible for making a good choice with that power.

Finally, try to find positive emotions that you resonate with or can embrace despite negativity. One positive emotion that can be particularly helpful to grasp is gratitude. Even when it feels like nothing is going right and nothing is okay, there is something to be grateful for. As cliche as it is, you have a roof over your head, someone who loves you, food, water, and other necessities like that. You have support. You have health. I'm not saying that you can never allow yourself to feel negativity; in fact, you *should* allow yourself to feel negative emotions. But rather than wrapping yourself up in those negative emotions, find the strength to look at the brighter side for a few moments and know that all is not bad.

MINDFULNESS

Another option that you have for improving your mental health and emotional well-being is mindfulness. Being mindful means being in the here and now, appreciating the present moment without judgment. It's simple but effective. Mindfulness encourages appreciation of the present, mental and emotional peace, and so much more, making it a vital skill for anyone to develop. Mindfulness can intertwine with IF, exercise, and general self-improvement as well. Some fantastic ways to develop your skill of mindfulness include

- **Gratitude:** Mindfulness and gratitude often go hand in hand. You can practice mindfulness through gratitude by taking a few moments to be appreciative of the things that you have that make life wonderful. I always recommend a gratitude journal for this. Take a few minutes every night to mindfully write down three to five things for which you are grateful. Over time, you'll become more and more positive—it really works!

- **Body check-ins:** You can bring mindfulness to even the most hectic of days by taking a few minutes to check in with your body. Your body often understands something you are going through before your mind does, so mindfulness can be a good way to check in with how you feel. Furthermore, body check-ins are a good method of grounding yourself in the present moment.

- **Focus on the heart:** Your heartbeat is one of the few things that will always be with you. Wherever you go and whoever you are with, you will have a heartbeat. You can focus on your heartbeat or the feeling of your pulse as a method to draw you to the present. This is especially effective if you feel like you are trapped in your head or need something simple to bring yourself to the present. You can hold your hand over your heart, check your pulse via your wrist, or even visualize the beating motion of your heart in your mind's eye.

- **Five senses:** A common therapeutic tactic involves engaging all five of your senses for present-moment awareness. You can try this tactic for yourself and experience the same soothing benefits that those in therapy achieve. To perform this activity, simply observe five things you can see, four you can touch, three you can hear, two you can smell, and one you can taste. Really allow yourself to be in the moment as you do this.

- **Mindful breathing:** Another way you can work with mindfulness is by breathing mindfully. To do this, simply start with an inhale. Pay attention to how the air feels entering your body and traveling through your airways. Pay attention to how it fills your lungs and how the air helps your belly to expand. Hold the air in for a moment before exhaling in a controlled manner, allowing yourself to track and feel the sensations of your breath leaving your body. Repeat this a few times until you feel present and at peace.

- **Thought observation:** Another method of mindfulness, one commonly considered to be a form of meditation, is to simply observe your thoughts without judgment. To engage with this, start by practicing mindful breathing, inhaling and exhaling with awareness. Then, simply relax. As thoughts come into your head, notice them, as if you are saying, "Hi there, I notice you."

Whether the thoughts are positive or negative, allow them to flow through your mind, noticing and releasing each butterfly of thought without criticism.

- **Mindful eating:** Mindful eating is a great way to appreciate your food and to avoid rushing through meals or stressing yourself out further due to considering eating to be just another chore. For details on how you can intertwine mindfulness and eating, feel free to refer back to Chapter 5!

- **Active listening:** The last tip that I have for you is to practice active listening. How often do you "listen" to someone and it goes in one ear and out of the other? You probably do this more often than you think! Try to actively listen to what someone is saying, allowing each word and sentence they speak to be a mindful consideration of yours. Avoid planning what you will say next or thinking about something else while someone is speaking to you.

SLEEP

A final consideration that you must keep in mind for improved mental and emotional well-being is sleep. Sleep is far more important than most people realize. The amount *and* quality of sleep that you get matters. Without enough high-quality sleep, not only will your physical health suffer, but your mental health and mood will suffer, too. Further, good sleep is needed for the effects of IF to truly be beneficial.

There are two things that you can work with to improve your sleep duration and quality: environment and lifestyle. Some things that you can do to create an environment that is more conducive to proper sleeping habits include

- **Decluttering your sleeping area:** Sure, you cannot see clutter while you are asleep, but the clutter that surrounds your bed and exists within your room can impact your mental state before sleeping. By decluttering your sleeping area, you can come to feel outer peace that contributes, in turn, to inner peace.
- **Reducing light infiltration:** The best sleeping environments are ones where low or no light is allowed into the room during winding down and sleeping hours. This means putting up high-quality curtains, as well as refusing to sleep with a TV or computer on in your room. For any lighting needs, consider low light sources like a salt lamp.
- **Employing symmetry:** You probably have quite a few pieces of furniture in your bedroom. Something you can do to enhance peace and aesthetic quality—both aspects that can improve sleep—is to use those pieces to create as much symmetry as possible. While you might not have two of everything to balance the room out perfectly, placing an equal amount of items on each side of the room can help quite significantly.
- **Finding the right pillow:** The right pillow can make a world of difference, which is why it is important to have a good quality, supportive pillow that meets height and material needs for sleep.

- **Trying a new mattress:** If you are struggling to sleep at night, you might need a different mattress. As your body changes, your needs regarding how firm or soft a mattress should be might change as well. This is a good time to invest in a new mattress.
- **Repainting:** You can also try repainting your room to a color that is more soothing, like desaturated versions of your favorite colors.

Then, some lifestyle changes that you can make that will enhance how well and how long you sleep are

- **Pick a good temperature.** Ideally, your sleeping temperature should be somewhere between 60 and 67 degrees Fahrenheit, and sometimes lower depending on if you suffer from night sweats. A cool, but not cold, bedroom is more conducive to proper sleep because the body naturally associates low body temperature with sleeping.
- **Don't consume caffeine after 2 p.m.** Consuming caffeine too late in the day is just asking to have trouble falling or staying asleep. If you drink caffeine, stop yourself from having that extra afternoon coffee to save yourself trouble when it comes to bedtime.
- **Get some exercise.** We've talked extensively about how exercise regulates your body temperature and circadian rhythms. Make sure to incorporate exercise into your daily routine both for IF and sleep benefits.
- **Have a bedtime routine.** A bedtime routine should begin an hour before you plan to go to sleep. Bedtime

routines psychologically calm and prepare you for bed, and they also work on a physiological level as well. A nighttime routine for going to bed will signal to your body and mind alike that it is time to wind down, making it easier and easier for you to hit the hay every night.

- **Don't nap after early afternoon.** Just like caffeine consumption can make it hard to fall or stay asleep, naps can, too. If you like to take naps or need them for a boost of energy—I recommend exercise for that, but I digress—try to stick to napping earlier on in the day or avoid naps altogether. It'll be hard at first, but over time, you'll get used to staying awake.
- **Don't hit snooze.** Sleeping in too late can make it hard for you to sleep well at night. Plus, hitting snooze trains your brain to wake up later and have a more erratic sleep schedule, which is not conducive to a good night's sleep.

Summary Box

In order to manage your emotions, you must learn to manage

- stress through adequate coping mechanisms.
- emotional regulation through tactics that are empowering and healthy.
- sleeping through proper sleep hygiene practices that improve the quality and duration of your sleep.

Managing your emotions and taking care of your mental health and well-being are important for allowing you to achieve total wellness. As you dive into your journey, it's important to understand that intermittent fasting can impact mental health, and the advice provided in this chapter is key to helping you maintain well-being while practicing intermittent fasting. In the next and final chapter of this book, you'll uncover how you can embrace intermittent fasting as a lifestyle.

8

EMBRACING A HEALTHIER, HAPPIER LIFESTYLE

Your body holds deep wisdom. Trust in it. Learn from it. Nourish it. Watch your life transform and be healthy.

— BELLA BLEUE

This chapter marks the final chapter in our journey together, but I'm not going to leave you empty-handed when it comes to intuitively and successfully integrating IF as a part of your lifestyle. In this final chapter of the book, you will find various strategies for maintaining intermittent fasting as a sustainable part of your lifestyle, allowing you to achieve long-term health benefits. This is the key to leading a happy, healthier life thanks to every skill you've picked up so far, so you won't want to skip out!

MAKING IF A LIFESTYLE

Now that you have all of the skills presented to you in the first seven chapters of the book, you have the power to turn those lessons into a foolproof plan for making IF a lifestyle—one that is infallible in the face of conflict or challenge. Some of the main skills you've gained involve personalizing fasting strategies, exercising, balancing nutrition, and taking care of your mental health. How can these considerations mesh together when it comes to making IF a lifestyle?

For starters, it is important to consider the impact one element has on the other elements. While it can be easier to think about fasting, exercise, nutrition, and mental health as separate elements with unique considerations, the fact of the matter is that each of these aspects plays a role as one component of what makes up you. In other words, it is beneficial to recognize that all elements impact all other elements.

Therefore, when it comes to making intermittent fasting and wellness a lifestyle, the considerations you make when it comes to your lifestyle have to be made with all other aspects in mind. It might seem great to have your fasting days on Tuesday and Thursday during a 5:2 fast, but if your only days to workout are Thursdays and Fridays, you know you get less sleep due to work on Monday nights, and you have zero time for healthy cooking on any of those days, maybe you should rework some things.

To make sense of conflicting scheduling, it can be a good idea to create a chart. Have seven columns, one for each day of the week, and 24 rows representing each hour of the day. Then, using different colors, outline when the best times and days would be for different lifestyle elements discussed in the book. Consider overlaps and nonnegotiable times before making a schedule. This will prevent you from fasting on days where you are low on energy and cannot fuel your body, or from exercising on days you are doing an intense fast.

Additionally, it is important that you realize that while exercise has rest days, no lifestyle has resting days. You might not exercise or even fast every day of the week, but you should still be following meal plans, eating balanced meals, getting enough sleep, engaging with emotional management, and more. You might not be fasting, but you are still in a *fasting cycle* even when you are in an active feeding window.

I tell you this because one of the biggest mistakes that people make is completely quitting their positive habits on days when they are not doing one of them. You do not have to do everything every day for it to be a success—keep this in mind as you form a lifestyle from IF and related habits.

It's also vital to come to terms with the fact that progress is not linear. One of the reasons so many people give up on their New Year's resolutions is that they miss a day or find themselves discouraged and quit. The realization that missing a day is not equivalent to failure is a positive one. Much like a New Year's resolution can still succeed if you miss one day of a habit, your IF journey can succeed even if you break a fast, forget you are fasting, overeat, or miss your exercise. Do not give up on a lifestyle journey because of a mistake!

Following IF Plans During a Busy Day

When it comes to taking intermittent fasting from a mere interest to a lifestyle, one of the biggest obstacles can be the challenges presented by a busy day. When you have so much going on in a day, food-related or not, it can be hard to fast consistently, break fasts at the right times, start fasts when they are meant to begin, and more. I definitely understand how these challenges can seem like obstacles!

Thankfully, just a few pieces of advice can make fasting during a busy day in your life seem more do-able:

- You can skip lunch during a fast and still take a lunch break. Sometimes, people misconstrue fasting during lunch as implying that they cannot take a lunch break period; that's not at all the case. During your lunch break, you can take some time to go for a walk, engage in mindfulness, journal, or even watch an episode of your favorite show. Do not think that your lunch break is confined to *eating* lunch.
- Try to avoid overcomplicating things. Asking yourself all sorts of "what if" questions can make fasting seem impossible. Just try it, and as obstacles meet you, be proactive in planning how you can overcome them. You do not have to account for every possible outcome before you can begin!
- Plan your fasting schedule around your work habits. If you need to, revisit Chapter 4, where we mentioned how you can personalize your fasting schedule and needs to fit in with work. You can make fasting fit into

your work schedule if you really want to. For example, if you *have* to eat at work for some reason, 5:2 fasting allows for a nice lunch at work and normal eating for most of the days in a week.

Fasting During the Holidays

Another reason that people say they cannot possibly make intermittent fasting a full-fledged lifestyle is because of the holidays. Especially in America, many of the holidays are known as times to eat a lot of food. Many people even *expect* that others eat large amounts of food on holidays, and such an expectation can feel power-stripping.

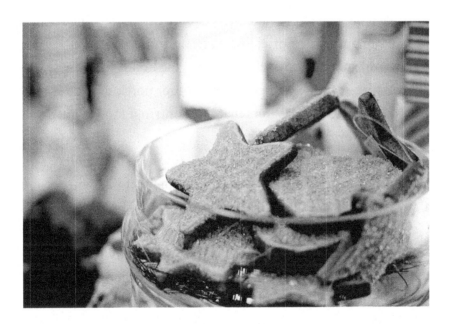

You can keep up your fasting habits during the holidays if you

- **Plan ahead.** Everyone knows when holiday celebrations are approaching, so you have no reason you cannot plan ahead. Even if it means changing your fasting schedule up a bit, you can plan around family social events that necessitate eating. You can also shift your fasting windows to account for travel, time zones, and more.
- **Make strategic food choices.** Many holiday foods are calorically dense, but you can make smart choices by going for vegetables, bringing healthier dishes to share, and having a small meal beforehand that is filling— allowing you to enjoy holiday food without needing to fill up on high-calorie, low-nutrient food.
- **Avoid snacking.** Snacking during the holidays often involves candies and chocolate, bigger portions for snacks, and other habits that can contribute to weight gain or breaking a fast early.
- **Let people know ahead of time.** You should make it a point to let people know ahead of time that you will be fasting or on a diet during the holidays. Be prepared to handle questions and misconceptions, and always stand up for yourself about your health. You can invite others to participate as well, but definitely allow them to make their own decisions about it.

BUILDING YOUR SUPPORT NETWORK

Life is boring and sad without companions to keep us company. Companionship and a strong support network are necessary for overall life satisfaction, and it can also make integrating intermittent fasting into your lifestyle easier. A support network is important for many reasons:

- **Encouragement:** When you have a support network that understands what your goals and aspirations are, especially if they have similar aspirations of their own, you can seek encouragement from them. When the road gets challenging, or you need an extra push in the right direction, your support group will be there for you.
- **Accountability:** A support network is a wonderful way to keep yourself accountable. Upon sharing your goals with others who are motivated to help you achieve them, you will be held accountable by them. You can share progress reports, challenges, and victories with one another for further support.
- **Advice:** Asking for advice is a million times easier when you have a support network by your side who knows what you are going through. With a support network of those on a similar journey, you can share stories and experiences with one another, learning from each other as you go.
- **Emotional support:** Support networks are a mind-blowing source of support when things feel too hard or even impossible. It's a support network that will

encourage you to pick yourself up, dust yourself off, and keep trying.

A support network will keep you on the right track for making major lifestyle changes, and that includes the integration of intermittent fasting. Even if someone does not participate in intermittent fasting or dieting of any kind, you can still include them within your support network. Some of the best ways to build and maintain a support network include

- **Sustaining current relationships:** One of the first things that you should do involves the prioritization of existing or past relationships. Take the time to reach out to people who you are friends with or were friends with in the past and lost touch with. Emphasize these connections and let them know you are forming your support network. Talk openly about your IF journey, but do not make others feel pressured to participate.
- **Looking for support online:** There are hundreds of places online to look for support networks, especially for something as common as intermittent fasting. You can look for local support networks, clubs, and groups using digital avenues, or you can join online support networks that stay on the web. Reddit, Facebook, and other social platforms typically have dozens of groups and circles dedicated to topics like IF.
- **Being open to others:** Make sure that you are not closing yourself off to other people. Just like you have to reach out to other people, people should feel like they can reach out to you. Post online that you are

looking for an IF buddy or group, and make sure that your message boxes are open (and that you check them regularly). Strive to be an empathetic person that real-life peers consider safe to confide in, and you'll naturally accumulate supportive friends that way as well.

- **Knowing when it is not working out:** Not every connection we make works out. It's important to identify when a connection is no longer worth your time so that you can avoid committing time, effort, and energy to someone who cannot or will not reciprocate it, or that you just do not have chemistry with. If someone makes you feel unheard or unseen, disrespects your opinions, or otherwise indicates that they do not value you, it is time to drop the connection.

At the end of the day, while intermittent fasting as a lifestyle can totally be a solo affair, connecting with others can truly make a world of difference. If you are really struggling to connect with others over similar interests and lifestyle decisions, you cannot go wrong with starting a blog or social page dedicated to your journey. That will amass followers and friends similar to you, with whom you can then bond!

EVOLVING WITH AGE

Before sending you off into the world to form this lifestyle, the last thing that I want to talk with you about is evolving with age. For many women, age is daunting; it is a creeping monster that aims to suck the life out of you, ruining everything you've gained and earned. Well, I'm here to tell you that a mentality like this is not only able to be defeated, but it is all in your head. You have the capacity to change how you consider age for enhanced satisfaction with your life, and it all starts with a few changes in your habits and how you think.

For example, in order to allow yourself to evolve as you age, you have to set achievable goals. Goals are good for everyone to have because they serve as a primary source of motivation; however, goals are especially important as you age because they provide some much-needed direction during a time in your life when things may feel particularly stagnant. Besides setting goals for health and intermittent fasting, you can also set goals pertaining to

- **Hobbies:** You can set goals that surround developing new hobbies, getting back into old hobbies, or perfecting skills that you already have.
- **Learning:** It's never too late to commit to learning a new skill, language, subject, and so on.
- **Career:** You can make major career advances or changes at any age.
- **Finance:** Savings goals are achievable at any age as well, and you have the opportunity to save up for that splurge item you've been wanting!

And much more. So long as a goal is attainable and gets you closer to who you want to be or what you want to have, you are on the right track.

In addition, evolving with age involves the development of self-awareness. Self-awareness refers to being aware not only of what you think and do, but also of why you think and do those things—including your motivations, intentions, biases, and inner workings. In order to develop self-awareness, I suggest keeping a journal and picking up the habit of writing in it daily. Every week, go back and look over your entries to see if you notice patterns, changes, or developments in the "how" and "why" of your thinking. You should also regularly question your beliefs, understanding why you feel a certain way or act how you do. Enhanced self-awareness makes you a stronger person who can grow as you age.

Being holistic about your overall lifestyle decisions is another change that can improve your satisfaction with life after the age of 50. Holistic, in this case, means ensuring that your efforts for growth don't just include one method or approach. For example, a holistic approach to wellness through intermittent fasting involves not just fasting, but nutrition, exercise, mental wellness, and more. Holistic approaches are better because they improve many aspects of your life all at once, and this holistic mindset is one that you can apply to every part of your life.

You should also learn to embrace your imperfections. 50 is far too old to be worried about something as silly as wrinkles, a loud laugh, goofy mistakes in daily life, or simply human error. All of these are signs that you have lived a vibrant life and are human, which is the most beautiful part of being alive. If everyone was perfect, the world would be quite a dull place! Learn to embrace your imperfections for a happier life. You can embrace imperfections by simply acknowledging them without judgment through mindfulness. They exist; they aren't good or bad.

Furthermore, you can create new habits for the new chapter in your life. What is one thing you've always wanted to do on a daily basis? Why not start doing it now? Starting new positive habits is a great way to signify a new chapter in your life and give it a special touch. Your life isn't ending because you've turned 50; a new chapter is just beginning, and you have so many years to write out the details! You can form habits pertaining to morning or evening routines, treating yourself to lunch, going on a date with yourself, spending time with your partner, and much more to make life especially meaningful.

Beyond that, there's no reason you can't just forget about your age altogether. There's no reason to say, "I can't do that, I'm 50!" Wear what you want, enjoy what you enjoy, participate in the hobbies that bring you satisfaction, and take advantage of all that life has to offer. So many women allow life to end at 50 simply because they view age as a sign to stop having fun. Whatever you do, don't let that be your experience, and you'll be so much happier for it in the end.

While age can be a frightening thing, bringing about new changes and obstacles, it's also an invitation to start over with new lifestyle choices and make your life yours once more. You don't have to give up on health or happiness at 50, or even 60, 70, or 80! Intermittent fasting is just one of the ways that you can embrace age; by implementing IF into your lifestyle, you are one step closer to embracing the fact that life is a continuing story with many chapters and not one long book that has ended on your 50th birthday. It's all about the lifestyle changes that you make today that pave your future—you decide what that road looks like.

FINAL REFLECTIONS: JOURNALING PROMPTS

Now that we are at the end of the journey, it is a good idea to take some time to reflect using the following journal prompts:

- Write about the personal reasons that led you to consider intermittent fasting as a part of your lifestyle. How do these reasons align with your values and long-term health goals? Reflecting on your motivations can reinforce your commitment to this lifestyle change.
- Describe the biggest challenges you have faced or anticipate facing in maintaining your intermittent fasting routine. How do these challenges affect your daily life and overall well-being? Consider strategies that could help you overcome these hurdles.
- Keep a record of your intermittent fasting journey. What patterns have you noticed? How has your body responded to the changes? Include both the physical and emotional aspects of your health. Use this space to celebrate small victories and contemplate any adjustments that might be beneficial.
- Beyond intermittent fasting, what other activities or habits contribute to your sense of wellness? List new habits you would like to adopt or current ones you want to enhance, such as exercise, mindfulness, or

adequate sleep, and how they fit into your healthier, happier lifestyle plan.

- How does intermittent fasting contribute to your happiness? Do you find that it impacts your mental clarity, energy levels, or mood? Write about the connection between your dietary habits and your mental health, and how you can nurture this connection moving forward.

Summary Box

You can still fast during the holidays if you

- Plan ahead for holiday celebrations.
- Make strategic food choices based on nutrient needs.
- Don't snack between meals.
- Let people know ahead of time that you plan to participate in fasting.

Closing out Chapter 8, it's important to understand that intermittent fasting is not just something you do one time and forget about. For the best benefits and results, it's a lifestyle that you have to commit to—one that you now have all of the tools for achieving. Thank you for coming with me on this journey—I know you're going to do amazing things with the opportunities you've gained!

CONCLUSION

As a woman above 50, or even a woman approaching 50, there are unique challenges that you face. Between mental changes like mood and energy and the physical changes that you're experiencing with your body, aging is taxing in every sense of the word. It can be hard to feel like a radiant, beautiful person with so many obstacles in the way.

But now, you have everything it takes to jump each and every hurdle that stops you from loving yourself, your body, and your life, all thanks to intermittent fasting. Intermittent fasting is a dynamic, flexible, safe, and incredible method of taking charge of your health without a single dime.

Throughout the course of this book, you've unearthed everything you need for the perfect F.A.S.T., all thanks to a unique four-part framework. You have a full understanding of what IF is, how it can be customized, how to stay safe, and everything you need to truly make IF your own and embrace the role it can play in your life.

Hundreds of women just like you have embraced the journey of intermittent fasting and achieved mind-blowing results, and it's your turn to follow their example. You have already taken an admirable step forward by completing this book; now, you just have to apply the skills. And you can contribute to helping other women find this resource by leaving a review (plus, I would appreciate it as well)!

You now have the tools to live a healthier life, and it's time to take action and make positive changes. It's not going to be an easy journey, but it will be worth it. Keep learning, growing, and challenging yourself. Good luck!

DID YOU ENJOY THE JOURNEY?
SHARE YOUR THOUGHTS!

Hey there, amazing reader!

You've just finished reading "The Ultimate Guide to Intermittent Fasting for Women Over 50." What a journey it's been, right? I hope you found it as enlightening and beneficial as I intended.

Now, I have a small but important favor to ask. If this book made a positive impact on your life, could you please share your experience with others? Your review could be the beacon of hope for another woman embarking on her intermittent fasting journey.

It's super simple and quick to do:

Please scan the QR Code below. Your insights and thoughts can truly make a difference.

Feel free to share what aspects you enjoyed most, what new things you learned, and how this book has helped you in your health journey.

Your words have the power to motivate another woman over 50 to embrace a healthier lifestyle, gain more energy, and feel empowered. This small gesture can have a huge impact.

Thank you for joining me on this adventure and for helping to guide others. You're fantastic!

Kevin Sterling

P.S. - Knowledge is most powerful when shared. If you know someone who could benefit from this guide, don't hesitate to pass it on. Together, we can make a positive change in the lives of many women over 50. Let's spread the wisdom!

REFERENCES

A dietitian's no-nonsense guide to fighting emotional eating. (n.d.). Houston Methodist. https://www.houstonmethodist.org/blog/articles/2020/dec/ a-dietitians-no-nonsense-guide-to-fighting-emotional-eating/

Bhirani, R. (2022, March 11). *Follow these 5 thumb rules to make the most of intermittent fasting for weight loss*. Healthshots. https://www.healthshots.com/ healthy-eating/nutrition/intermittent-fasting-tips-5-things-you-must- do-right-for-weight-loss/

Bleue, B. (n.d.). *Quote*. In Geurin, Lori. (2021). *42 powerful intermittent fasting quotes to spark your motivation*. Wellness for Life. https://lorigeurin.com/ intermittent-fasting-quotes/

Can you drink water during intermittent fasting? here's the answer. (2023, May 13). HealthifyMe. https://www.healthifyme.com/blog/water-during-intermit tent-fasting/#:~:

The connection between menopause & belly fat. (n.d.). UH Hospitals. https:// www.uhhospitals.org/blog/articles/2023/08/the-connection-between- menopause-and-belly-fat

Damianou, P. (2023, August 28). *Intermittent fasting: 10 common mistakes!* Vita4you Blog. https://www.vita4you.gr/blog-vita4you/en/item/intermit tent-fasting-10-common-mistakes.html

de Rochefoucauld, F. (n.d.). *Quote*. In Geurin, Lori. (2021). *42 powerful intermittent fasting quotes to spark your motivation*. Wellness for Life. https:// lorigeurin.com/intermittent-fasting-quotes/

The definitive guide to healthy eating in your 50s and 60s. (2021, September 20). Healthline. https://www.healthline.com/nutrition/healthy-eating-50s- 60s#nutrients-foods

DeSilva, D. (2021, July 20). *Nutrition as we age: healthy eating with the dietary guidelines*. Health.gov. https://health.gov/news/202107/nutrition-we-age- healthy-eating-dietary-guidelines

Eckelkamp, S. (2020, January 21). *Intermittent fasting? here's the right way to break your fast*. Mindbodygreen. https://www.mindbodygreen.com/arti cles/intermittent-fasting-heres-right-way-to-break-your-fast

Emotional regulation skills: learn how to manage your emotions. (2022, April 6). Psych Central. https://psychcentral.com/health/emotional-regulation

Exercise rest day: benefits, importance, tips, and more. (2019, August 7). Healthline. https://www.healthline.com/health/exercise-fitness/rest-day#signs-you-need-rest

5 reasons women over 50 need to exercise more. (2020, November 3). Curves. https://www.curves.com/blog/move/5-reasons-women-over-50-need-to-exercise-more

Geurin, Lori. (2021). *42 powerful intermittent fasting quotes to spark your motivation.* Wellness for Life. https://lorigeurin.com/intermittent-fasting-quotes/

Gunnars, K. (2020, January 1). *6 popular ways to do intermittent fasting.* Healthline. https://www.healthline.com/nutrition/6-ways-to-do-intermittent-fasting

Haas, E. (n.d.). *Quote.* In Geurin, Lori. (2021). *42 powerful intermittent fasting quotes to spark your motivation.* Wellness for Life. https://lorigeurin.com/intermittent-fasting-quotes/

Health benefits of intermittent fasting (and tips for making it work). (n.d.). UCLA Health. https://www.uclahealth.org/news/health-benefits-of-intermittent-fasting-and-tips-for-making-it-work

Hormones as you age. (n.d.). Rush. https://www.rush.edu/news/hormones-you-age#:~

How to build a strong support network. (n.d.). Suicide Call Back Service. https://www.suicidecallbackservice.org.au/mental-health/how-to-build-a-strong-support-network/

How to choose the best fasting diet that works for your metabolism. (n.d.). Lumen. https://www.lumen.me/blog/nutrition/find-out-which-intermittent-fasting-schedule-will-work-for-you

How to exercise safely during intermittent fasting. (2023, May 4). Healthline. https://www.healthline.com/health/how-to-exercise-safely-intermittent-fasting#takeaway

How to personalize intermittent fasting for your clients. (n.d.). LinkedIn. https://www.linkedin.com/pulse/how-personalize-intermittent-fasting-your-clients-ashley-koff-rd/

How to start over in life at 50: it's never too late. (n.d.). BetterUp. https://www.betterup.com/blog/how-to-start-over-in-life-at-50

The importance of good nutrition. (n.d.). Tufts Medicare Preferred. https://www.

tuftsmedicarepreferred.org/healthy-living/importance-good-nutrition#:~:text=Good%20nutrition%20can%20help%3A

Instead of calories, you should track this key health metric. (n.d.). CNET. https://www.cnet.com/health/nutrition/instead-of-calories-you-should-track-this-key-health-metric/

Is fasting safe for women over 50? An OB/GYN weighs in. (2023, March 31). Mindbodygreen. https://www.mindbodygreen.com/articles/intermittent-fasting-for-women-over-50

Johns Hopkins Medicine. (2021). *Intermittent fasting: What is it, and how does it work?* Johns Hopkins Medicine. https://www.hopkinsmedicine.org/health/wellness-and-prevention/intermittent-fasting-what-is-it-and-how-does-it-work

khore. (2016, November 23). *Strength training for women over 50.* Australian Fitness Academy. https://www.fitnesseducation.edu.au/blog/personal-training/strength-training-for-women-over-50/

Living an intermittent fasting lifestyle. (n.d.). https://stoughtonhealth.com/wp-content/uploads/Living-an-intermittent-fasting-lifestyle-presentation-7.15.2020.pdf

Loncaric, S. (2018, February 6). *6 benefits of cardio workouts for over 50 women.* Women Living Well after 50. https://www.womenlivingwellafter50.com.au/cardio-workouts-for-women-over-50/

Macronutrients for the older adult. (n.d.). StrongerLife. https://www.strongerlifehq.com/blog/macros-for-the-older-adult

Madwire, D. (2020, August 21). *Other ways to track your progress besides the scale.* Life Wellness Center. https://www.lifewellnesscenter.net/weight-loss/other-ways-to-track-your-progress-besides-the-scale/#:~

Medicine, G. F. I. G. (2022, February 4). *Intermittent fasting: Benefits, how it works, and is it right for you?* Good-Food. https://health.ucdavis.edu/blog/good-food/intermittent-fasting-benefits-how-it-works-and-is-it-right-for-you/2022/02

Menopause & depression, mood changes. (2020). Menopause.org. https://www.menopause.org/for-women/menopauseflashes/mental-health-at-menopause/depression-menopause

Mindfulness matters. (2017, June 28). NIH News in Health. https://newsinhealth.nih.gov/2012/01/mindfulness-matters

Nazish, N. (n.d.). *10 intermittent fasting myths you should stop believing.* Forbes.

https://www.forbes.com/sites/nomanazish/2021/06/30/10-intermittent-fasting-myths-you-should-stop-believing/?sh=7454d28d335b

New data on how intermittent fasting affects female hormones. (n.d.). UIC. https://ahs.uic.edu/kinesiology-nutrition/news/new-data-on-how-intermittent-fasting-affects-female-hormones/

Obama, M. (n.d.) *Quote.* In Geurin, Lori. (2021). *42 powerful intermittent fasting quotes to spark your motivation.* Wellness for Life. https://lorigeurin.com/intermittent-fasting-quotes/

Robinson, L. (2020, October). *Mindful eating.* HelpGuide. https://www.helpguide.org/articles/diets/mindful-eating.htm

Sadhguru. (n.d.). *Quotes.* In Geurin, Lori. (2021). *42 powerful intermittent fasting quotes to spark your motivation.* Wellness for Life. https://lorigeurin.com/intermittent-fasting-quotes/

Strength training exercises for women over 50: all you need to know. (n.d.). Nutrisense. https://www.nutrisense.io/blog/strength-training-for-women-over-50

Stress management stress basics. (n.d.). Mayo Clinic. https://www.mayoclinic.org/healthy-lifestyle/stress-management/basics/stress-basics/hlv-20049495#:~

Warm-up and cool-down. (n.d.). NHS Inform. https://www.nhsinform.scot/healthy-living/keeping-active/before-and-after-exercise/warm-up-and-cool-down/#:~

WebMD Editorial Contributors. (2021, September 27). *What to know about intermittent fasting for women after 50.* WebMD. https://www.webmd.com/healthy-aging/what-to-know-about-intermittent-fasting-for-women-after-50

Why maintaining a healthy weight is important as you get older. (n.d.). Beth and Howard Braver MD. https://www.bethandhowardbravermd.com/blog/why-maintaining-a-healthy-weight-is-important-as-you-get-older

Wirth, J. (2022, October 25). *The most important nutrients as you age—and where to find them.* Forbes Health. https://www.forbes.com/health/healthy-aging/important-nutrients-as-you-age/

Working out while intermittent fasting. (n.d.). Atkins. https://www.atkins.com/how-it-works/library/articles/6-things-to-know-about-intermittent-fasting-and-working-out

IMAGE REFERENCES

congerdesign. (n.d.). *Noodles, rice, potatoes* [Image]. Pixabay. https://pixabay. com/photos/noodles-rice-potatoes-food-pasta-516635/

dbreen. (n.d.). *Vegetables, fruits, food* [Image]. Pixabay. https://pixabay.com/ photos/vegetables-fruits-food-ingredients-1085063/

Einladung_zum_Essen. (n.d.). *Breakfast, healthy, hummus* [Image]. Pixabay. https://pixabay.com/photos/breakfast-healthy-hummus-spread-1804457/

FunkyFocus. (n.d.). *Hourglass, time, monk* [Image]. Pixabay. https://pixabay. com/photos/hourglass-time-monk-buddhist-1875812/

IamNotPerfect. (n.d.). *Water, glass, tilted* [Image]. Pixabay. https://pixabay.com/ photos/water-glass-tilted-clear-drink-2315559/

JanBaby. (n.d.). *Heart, beat, heart beat* [Image]. Pixabay. https://pixabay.com/ photos/heart-beat-heart-beat-heartbeat-2211180/

JillWellington. (n.d.). *Christmas cookies, xmas, Christmas* [Image]. Pixabay. https://pixabay.com/photos/christmas-cookies-xmas-christmas-2918172/

silviarita. (n.d.). *Women, girlfriends, nature* [Image]. Pixabay. https://pixabay. com/photos/women-girlfriends-nature-walk-3394510/

stevepb. (n.d.). *Physiotherapy, weight training, dumbbells* [Image]. Pixabay. https://pixabay.com/photos/physiotherapy-weight-training-595529/

StockSnap. (n.d.). *Woman, jogging, running* [Image]. Pixabay. https://pixabay. com/photos/woman-jogging-running-exercise-2592247/

Made in the USA
Las Vegas, NV
25 January 2024

84787538R00095